Outsider Art and Psychoanalytic Psychiatry

Outsider Art and Psychoanalytic Psychiatry is a study of psychiatric institutes and psychiatric violence as seen through art created by the inhabitants of a psychiatric hospital.

Cosimo Schinaia explores the history of the Cogoleto Psychiatric Hospital, now abandoned, and how its architecture and ideology influenced treatment of the patients who lived there. At the book's core is an in-depth historical, anthropological, and psychoanalytical study of the "Nativity of Fools," a large art installation constructed from 1980 to 1984 by patients, nurses, and psychiatrists, representing their everyday lives in the asylum. Schinaia's understanding of the scenes considers questions of nostalgia, isolation, privacy, and freedom and reflects on the risks of institutionalised segregation. The book proposes original psychoanalytic reflections on the subject of the obsolescence of psychiatric hospitals and treating mental suffering without institutionalising people.

This book will be of great interest to psychoanalysts in practice and in training, psychiatrists, psychologists, social workers, and nurses as well as readers interested in outsider art, Arte Povera, and the history of psychiatric institutions and contemporary psychiatry.

Cosimo Schinaia is a training and supervising psychoanalyst of SPI (Italian Psychoanalytic Society) and a full member of IPA (International Psychoanalytical Association), working in private practice in Genoa. He was formerly the director of the Cogoleto Psychiatric Hospital (Genoa) and of the Mental Health Centre of Central Genoa. He has published many scientific papers on psychoanalysis and psychiatry in Italian and international journals and edited books. His books include *On Paedophilia* (Routledge, 2010), also published in Italian, French, Spanish, Portuguese, Polish, German, Russian and Greek, *Psychoanalysis and Architecture: The Inside and the Outside* (Routledge, 2016), also published in Italian, Spanish and French, and *Psychoanalysis and Ecology: The Unconscious and the Environment* (Routledge, 2022), also published in Italian, French, Spanish, Russian, Greek and Portuguese.

Outsider Art and Psychoanalytic Psychiatry: The "Nativity of Fools" at the Cogoleto Psychiatric Hospital is published in Italian and Spanish.

Psychoanalytic Ideas and Applications Series
Series Editor: Silvia Flechner

Outsider Art and Psychoanalytic Psychiatry

The "Nativity of Fools" at the Cogoleto Psychiatric Hospital

Cosimo Schinaia

Translated by Giuseppe Lo Dico and Kathryn Haralambous

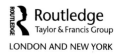

Routledge
Taylor & Francis Group

LONDON AND NEW YORK

Designed cover image: © Photograph by Margherita Loewy

First published in English 2024
by Routledge
4 Park Square, Milton Park, Abingdon, Oxon OX14 4RN

and by Routledge
605 Third Avenue, New York, NY 10158

Routledge is an imprint of the Taylor & Francis Group, an informa business

© 2024 Cosimo Schinaia

Published in Italian by Alpes Italia srl (2018)
© Il presepe dei folli, (2018)
First published in 2018 by Alpes Italia srl. All rights reserved.
Original title: Il Presepe dei folli

British Library Cataloguing-in-Publication Data
A catalogue record for this book is available from the British Library

ISBN: 978-1-032-46451-0 (hbk)
ISBN: 978-1-032-46450-3 (pbk)
ISBN: 978-1-003-38172-3 (ebk)

DOI: 10.4324/9781003381723

Typeset in Palatino
by MPS Limited, Dehradun

To Dario De Martis and Fausto Petrella, my guides and mentors.

To all the women and men who have lived in a psychiatric hospital.

To all the women and men who will never live in a psychiatric hospital.

Contents

Series Editor's Foreword

The International Psychoanalytic Association Publications Committee continues with the present volume of the series "Psychoanalytic Ideas and Applications."

These series aim to focus on the scientific output of significant authors whose works are outstanding contributions to the development of the psychoanalytic field.

We aim to share these ideas with the psychoanalytic community and related professionals of other disciplines that could expand their communication and generate a productive exchange to get more knowledge in this field.

The Publications Committee is pleased to publish the book *The Nativity of Fools at Cogoleto Psychiatric Hospital* by Cosimo Schinaia.

Dr. Cosimo Schinaia is a psychiatrist and training and supervising psychoanalyst of the Italian Psychoanalytic Society and a full member of the IPA, working in private practice in Genoa. He was the director of the Cogoleto Psychiatric Hospital (Genoa) and the Mental Health Centre of Central Genoa. He published many scientific papers on psychoanalysis and psychiatry in Italian and other languages and many books. *The Nativity of Fools* at Cogoleto Psychiatric Hospital is published in Italian and Spanish.

The author refers that after 21 years, the book is published again with a new foreword for the 40th anniversary of the Basaglia Law, which led to the closedown of all the psychiatric hospitals in Italy. After many years of silence, the book proposes an original psychoanalytic reflection on the obsolescence of psychiatric hospitals again. It warns against the risks that the inhuman idea of institutionalised segregation can take place in those new psychiatric services planned and designed as antithetical to the concept of a psychiatric hospital.

The author states: "In a long, winding, and tight corridor of an abandoned ward in the old Psychiatric Hospital of Cogoleto, near Genoa, there is a sequence of scenes representing the key moments of the life inside the Asylum. The so-called 'Nativity scene of fools' is more than 500 square meters. It clearly (and nostalgically) reconstructs the history of the old psychiatric hospital, the abandonment and segregation of its patients, the pediatric ward, the places of the pseudo-therapeutic violence, the farming colony, and the obliged occupations passed off as ergotherapy. The last scene represents Genoa, the city where it could be possible to live with other people and not be forcefully separated."

The book is written by assuming that a particular piece of artwork known as the Nativity scene of the former psychiatric hospital of Cogoleto is a fil rouge for discussing the limits of a specific idea of institutional psychiatry and for showing what psychoanalysis can offer as concrete solutions to some unresolvable problems of the psychiatric hospitals.

The text offers numerous aspects of this problematic situation: the historical, the psychoanalytic, the psychiatric, the social critical register, and the narrative.

The author can trace the historical and artistic roots of the Nativity scene in the psychiatric hospital can be traced back to both the Eighteen Century Neapolitan Nativity scenes (characterised by an almost absolute realism), the Nativity scenes of the Provence, depicted by different settings with puppets (santons). In the Nativity scene of Cogoleto, nothing is reparatory or consolatory. The pain is immediately perceivable, and the patient's condition is revealed without any defensive mask.

Cogoleto's Asylum, from its origins to its closure, summarises the history of Italian psychiatric hospitals; reading this book sensitises us about the past and present difficulties regarding mental health and its vicissitudes.

Silvia Flechner
Series Editor
Chair, IPA Publications Committee

But when from a long-distant past nothing subsists, after the people are dead, after the things are broken and scattered, taste and smell alone, more fragile but more enduring, more unsubstantial, more persistent, more faithful, remain poised a long time, like souls, remembering, waiting, hoping, amid the ruins of all the rest; and bear unflinchingly, in the tiny and almost impalpable drop of their essence, the vast structure of recollection.

Marcel Proust, *Swann's Way*, 1913.

What am I in the eyes of most people? A nonentity or an oddity or a disagreeable person — someone who has and will have no position in society, in short a little lower than the lowest.

Very well — assuming that everything is indeed like that, then through my work I'd like to show what there is in the heart of such an oddity, such a nobody.

This is my ambition, which is based less on resentment than on love in spite of everything, based more on a feeling of serenity than on passion.

Vincent van Gogh, *Letter to His Brother Theo*,
on or about July 21, 1882.

Acknowledgements

I could have never imagined this book without the visionary idea and subsequent coordination and work of Tomaso Molinari. He was the head nurse who first had the idea of patients creating a big Nativity Scene at Cogoleto Psychiatric Hospital in Genoa, a *crèche* markedly different from the traditional ones, that represented the life of the asylum in its transition phase, when the old was dying in agony and the new was not still defined.

The craft skills and artistic sensibility of Bruno Galati, a gardener at the hospital, were also fundamental. He created most of the pottery, papier-mâché statuettes, and scenes. He transformed Molinari's memories and experiences in a piece of Arte Povera (poor art).[1] Later he became an important artist with a hyperrealist style and directed psychiatric rehabilitation projects at the hospital's pottery studio.

Further, I would like to thank all the patients and mental health workers who brought their skills, abilities, and memories to the Nativity Scene: each made an important contribution to the project.

A special thanks is reserved for the art historian Giovanna Rotondi Terminiello, who for decades tended to the artistic heritage of the Region of Liguria. She immediately recognised the historic and artistic merit of the piece and did her utmost to conserve it. So, too, I thank her for her afterword, in which she describes the present condition of the work of art.

I am deeply grateful to my mentor and lifelong friend Fausto Petrella for the openheartedness he expresses in his passionate and thought-provoking foreword.

I am grateful to Humberto Lorenzo Persano for his stimulating foreword to the Argentinian edition of this book.

I thank Francesco Barale, Tiziana Bastianini, Giorgio Bergami, Armando Besio, Natale Calderaro, Rocco Canosa, Lino Ciancaglini, Pietro Ciliberti, Carmelo Conforto, Giorgio Cosmacini, Luigi Ferrannini, Antonio Maria Ferro, Marie Antoinette Ferroni, Costantino Gilardi, Giuseppe Giunti, Vito Guidi, Piero Iozzia, Ezio Maria Izzo, Uliano Lucas, Angelo Magnano, Emilio Maura, Giovanni Meriana, Gianfranco Meterangelis, Bruno Orsini, Paolo Francesco Peloso, Mariangela PIrami, Pierluigi Politi, Adriano Sansa, and

Simone Vender. In different ways, each contributed to the conception and development of this book.

A tender and grateful thought is for Antonio Balletto, Giuseppe Berti Ceroni, Piera Bevilacqua, Aristo Ciruzzi, Michel David, Dario De Martis, Gilda De Simone, Antonio Drommi, Giovanni Franzoni, Roberto Ghirardelli, Giuseppe Menduni, Sergio Piro, Edoardo Sanguineti, Franco Sborgi, Antonio Slavich, Gian Soldi, and Gianfranco Vendemmiati, who are not here anymore.

I wish to remember those who joined forces to close down Cogoleto Psychiatric Hospital: Marco Barisone, Elisabetta Biancucci, Nicola Buogo, Orietta Cagnana, Luisa Ciammella, Maurizio Cristofanini, Maurizio Ferro, Camelia Jianu, Luigi Maccioni, Claudio Marcenaro, Antonio Pischedda, Olga Schiaffino, Claudia Traversa, Simona Traverso, Massimo Valeri, Cristina Valle, and all the mental health workers who made many efforts to propose alternatives to the psychiatric hospitals.

I also thank Professor Daniela Pittaluga, of the Polytechnic School at Genoa University, for her efforts in studying, conserving, and restoring the work of art; and Maurizio Gugliotta and Luca Nanni, whose association of volunteers continue to preserve the memory of those places and their stories.

My last and very special expression of gratitude is to Margherita Loewy, whose photographs lifted the Nativity Scene to come out of the grounds of a forgotten pavilion of an old psychiatric hospital and put it before the curious and moved eyes of many women and men.

Note

1 Arte Povera is an artistic movement created in contrast to traditional art. It rejects the techniques of traditional art in favour of "poor" materials such as soil, wood, iron, and rags. It aims to evoke the original linguistic structure of contemporary society. Another feature of Arte Povera is how it is installed: in deciding where to install a piece of such art, one considers the relationship between it and the environment.

Introduction to the English Edition

The Creation of the Nativity Scene

The Basaglia Law, or Law 180, which reformed Italy's psychiatric system and closed down all its psychiatric hospitals, was passed in 1978. However, it was only at the end of the 1990s that these places of exclusion and institutional violence were definitively shut.

During that in between time, in the early 1980s, some nurses and patients, supported by some physicians, planned and built a nativity scene which represented the lives and suffering and the hopes and dreams of the women and men internees at Cogoleto Psychiatric Hospital. Their nativity scene is larger than 500 square metres. They built it in the basement of a pavilion in which once there was a printing press. They finished it in 1984, after four years of hard and voluntary work.

A large group of institutionalised patients scavenged for the humble materials (branches, wire, old dishes, etc.) to build the work of art inside the psychiatric hospital. Bruno Galati, a young gardener at the hospital and talented craftsman, created the settings and statuettes. Unlike traditional nativity scenes, which last only during Christmas, this is a permanent installation and a memento with a strong ethical and aesthetic message.

To represent the misery suffered in a mental institution by creating a nativity scene is to be evocative: a nativity scene often holds a special place in our childhood memories. For many people, including many patients, it is a symbol of folk religion infused with the world of dreams and fairy tales.

Unlike similar artistic-artisanal representations, the Cogoleto Nativity Scene does not aim to comfort: the suffering is immediately visible, palpable, shared, and represented from different perspectives. There is no room for embellishment, compromise solutions, or defensive masks. An institutionalised world represented through paintings and scenes is an exceptional testament, a vivid document of the oppressive daily routines of the patients.

This unique nativity scene is also powerful because it serves cathartic and pedagogical functions, along with historic and documentary research and denunciation, and defence and self-observation.

Thanks to the first edition of this book in 1997, the Nativity Scene's statuettes went beyond the wall of the psychiatric hospital and held a wide appeal with the general public; they were featured in Italian newspapers and many popular, scientific, and cultural magazines.

The beautiful photographs of Margherita Loewy became icons of an outsider reality which deserved to be told and not repressed. They are both a testimony and a symbol of an invisible existential vitality that could be appreciated far beyond the visible edges.

For reparative, mysterious, and fascinating reasons, a phenomenon that appears to be impossible in harsh conditions—collective creativity and artistic production—occurred in an inhospitable environment, the psychiatric hospital, like a plant which can flourish in the desert. Perhaps this was a phenomenon unique in the world. It is a testimony to the extreme and heroic survival of the Self in a desert of human relationships.

Unfortunately, in spite of the promises of some politicians and administrators, today, after 35 years, the Nativity scene is abandoned. It is ruined, covered with dust, neglected. It remains in the basement of the same sad pavilion, an abandoned area for which there are no concrete or respectful projects of reuse. What had been lived and narrated as a symbol of a hope for emancipation, now seems a symbol of decay.

Its destiny parallels that of the hopes for the reutilisation of the 100 hectares of the psychiatric hospital's area. Many projects have been proposed for reusing this area, but none have come to fruition. Some were progressive, such as relocating the campus and botanical garden of the Faculty of Agricultural and Food Science of the University of Genoa.

After many years, I returned to visit the Nativity Scene along with the art historian Giovanna Rotondi Terminiello. Twenty years ago, she, as superintendent of cultural heritage of Liguria, and I, as director of the hospital, formed an association to protect, restore, and give value to important artworks produced in the hospital. For example, the painter Gino Grimaldi had been a patient at the hospital in the early 1900s: a canvas he created, which was displayed in the hospital's church, was restored, moved to an oratory in the city, and shown to the public in important exhibitions organised by the art critic Bianca Tosatti. But no one paid attention to the great Nativity scene. Invaded by rats, entire sections ripped off, its beautiful statues torn down. How is possible that so significant, original, and historically relevant artwork can have been forgotten? What about the promises of relocating the Nativity scene in a place where it can be restored and then protected, preserved, and exhibited?

Architectonic Thinking and Therapeutic Thinking

Even mental health services often appear to be covered by dust and neglected. In Italy they are often located in places not planned or designed for mental health, without an architectonic principle which considers the emotional and affective needs of the suffering people and their specific spatial needs (and, of course, the therapeutic needs of the health workers). Instead such places are often conceived, built, and furnished according to other functions. For example, spaces intended for social and administrative functions are often carelessly re-used. This lack of architectural thought relating to therapeutic thought often leads medical staff to receive patients in spaces that are anonymous, lifeless, and vague, and do not contain or promote socialisation. In such places suffering women and men become merely passive objects of therapy, restricted to partitioned spaces that prevent them from reconstructing the split-off parts of their selves and often maintain the splitting.

Throughout history, psychiatrists and architects have reflected on spaces for taking care of people who suffer, often from a paternalistic and authoritarian perspective. The psychiatric hospital was once a monolith characterised by grand and linear geometries. Based on the principles of Neoclassicism, it deployed symmetry as a symbol of order, equilibrium, and authority. In the history of the planning of psychiatric hospitals there is a shift from the phalanstery, based on Bentham's *Panopticon*, with its aim of absolute transparency and visual control, to Esquirol's Psychiatric Hospital (1938), for whom the psychiatric hospital was no mere therapeutic locale but a truly curative and healing device.

Jean-Étienne Dominique Esquirol designed the Charenton asylum with the architect Emile-Jacques Gilbert: he believed that designing a psychiatric hospital was not something that could be left only to architects. In opposition to both Bentham's *Panopticon* and Esquirol's asylum, there were isolated attempts to transform the psychiatric hospital into a sort of rural village. Examples include the Belgian city of Geel, with its early adoption of de-institutionalisation in psychiatric care, the widespread cottages system in England and the open-door model in Scotland (Maura and Peloso, 1999). Such spaces were conceived as dispersed settlements with separate pavilions surrounded by vegetation. The advantage was the promotion of outdoor work and living; the disadvantages, its far-flung location, and its autarchic and self-referential nature. Living and working outdoors is not enough to promote a cure and wellbeing. To make matter worse and to highlight the repression and exclusion that characterised the institution, the spaces were neatly subdivided to permit violence and constriction, although it was justified by hygienic-naturalistic intents. The fools were in one space, the psychiatrists in another one. They shut themselves off in their medical rooms and talked about the fools who were in distant wards. There was no possibility of meeting. If a meeting had to occur, it took place in medical rooms, not in the wings in which patients resided. Nurses entered these wings only for the time necessary to perform their functions; they found shelter in other, separate, and protected spaces, where they could avoid contact with the patients or, more precisely, avoid the risk of becoming "infected" with mental disease.

Today in the psychiatric wards the division of space is less defined but, at the same time, more differentiated. Near the wards we can find the nurses' and physicians' rooms, a small kitchen, etc. They can be seen as spaces for attenuating and suspending the anxiety over mental disease, where one can feel part of the "healthy" group and avoid a dangerous encounter with mental pain and disease.

Planning new therapy spaces should first consider the primary and secondary needs of patients and also these of health workers, their mental balance, and the defensive necessities emanating from extended and demanding contact with high levels of suffering. The planning of intermediate places and transitional spaces should avoid the construction of hidden and seemingly comforting (but actually anti-relational and isolating) refuges, similar to crypts in which anxiety cannot be avoided.

Hippocrates argued that healing depends also on external circumstances and structure of therapeutic places. Ancient Greek hospitals boasted beautiful architecture and spaces for acting and creating art. In the 15th century, in the introduction of his *De re aedificatoria*, Leon Battista Alberti wrote about the therapeutic function of architecture. Later, the Renaissance saw frescoed hospital walls and roofs. This continued. In the Age of Enlightenment physical and moral hygiene was stressed and therapeutic function was attributed to psychiatric architecture; under Modernism hospitals, summer camps, kitchens, and sanatoriums were built according to the principles of transparency and brightness. The *mens sana in corpore sano* (a sound mind in a sound body) in Juvenal's *Satire X* was transferred from the human body to the environment. However, it is worth noting that here the central place of the psychophysical balance was far from being recognised. In fact, from the Age of Enlightenment onward we invented many "health machines" for saving people. Further, the 20th century introduced architectural solutions for bringing forth the disinfectant properties of sunlight and hygiene products.

The spaces conceived according to this view follow a therapeutic logic that does not consider a possible integration between the disease to be eradicated and the person to be treated. According to this logic, the emotional distance from the patients and their disease is a consequence. We can even say that emotional neutrality is a prescription or a necessary condition of the therapeutic organisation. The same features of neutrality can be found in the hospital, in which the use of colours (generally, white, grey, green, or blue), material (generally, metal, or synthetic), lights, and finishing touches are in tune with hygiene and the quality of medical performance. The predominance of functional and hygienic dimensions obscures the possibility that the environment can promote interactive processes between people, therapeutic activities, and medical tools, and thus it does not allow for the recognition of the emotional influence of space over the patients and health workers.

The receiving environments cannot be based upon general, rationalising, or depersonalising models such as traditional hospitals and clinics. These models have their roots in strong cultural references such as Le Corbusier's *machine à habiter*. The rationale underlying the creation of this machine is the complete sanitisation of space and the predominant use of the colour white. Such spaces must be avoided because they can prevent if not outright censor conversation and can pose an insurmountable barrier to horizontal exchanges. These models do not allow the expression of emotions and feelings in any way (Schinaia, 2019).

Today it is not completely clear how the connection between psychosis and environment is conceived (this is of course due to the complex interrelations and the many causal factors at the basis of mental disease). In spite of this, we can say that there is a great lack of specific projects and plans (and also of appropriate economic investment) for places of therapy for mental disease, that is, places in which patients can be revitalised and recognised as persons and the therapeutic relationships can be protected.

On the one hand, the structures devoted to psychiatric disease need to be coherently integrated into the urban-fabric and thus should be in harmony and even be part of the urban landscape. This would replace the stigmatising image of the diversity of mental patients with comforting places that could help them return to life in the city. On the other hand, there are paltry few administrative and architectural models appropriate for the therapeutic needs of people who suffer; that is, few models propose personal, specific, and unique routes and trajectories capable of flexibly considering the need of being alone or isolated, of containing the confusion and the undifferentiated, or, on the contrary, of tolerating what is rigidly and defensively split off.

Thus, there is a need for specialised spaces with defined and recognisable architectures in which the communication about a therapeutic question and the proposal of a therapy or a form of assistance can be formalised and institutionalised. An example is the organisation of the room for the first appointment and individual or group therapy in mental health services. At the same time, this is strictly connected to the interstitial places,[1] those lacking a formal and codified language, open to informal, less hierarchical, and divisive communication, in which we can search for what lacks structure, meaning, or shape, what is not expressed. They are places in transition in the mind (Roussillon, 1988), in which the size of the rooms, the brightness of the environment, the colours of the walls, and the arrangement of the furniture are planned according to an unspecific and circumscribed therapeutic function. This demands an intermediate space between the everyday relationships and the specialised relationship, between the spontaneity of a meeting between people and the intentionality of the therapeutic setting.

This is not a proposal for completely reproducing the domestic environment in the new therapeutic setting, similarly to when a retirement home replicates the person's old bedroom back home. This is confusing and useless. This "Disneyland ideology" confuses a process of respectful care with a form of childhood entertainment and does not permit the elaboration of the loss of the home or the acceptance of a new life environment.

According to Anna Ferruta (2009), the institutional psychiatric architecture for the cure of the mental patients should be made of spatial-temporal constructions able to promote the development of lively relationships for both patients and mental institutions and to integrate beauty, creativity, participation, and individuality. Even in the therapeutic relationship, solid but strange buildings can be construed. Such buildings can become prisons in which mental life can languish and die. Even a very personal and not institutional architectural structure can be a prison, a false movement, the ideology of a movement, a container that has become a content and that does not allow any dialogue, contact, free meeting, approach, or departure.

It is objectively more difficult, but nonetheless more fascinating, to think about and then create avenues of real freedom and democracy which promote, support, and protect the passage from the inside to the outside and vice versa. These avenues must be designed as interconnected and intertwined and having rest stops or transitional spaces that permit one to become used to the new landscape, that facilitate the mourning of the old habits in a sober way, without strong breaks, in respect of the time required to do this. This need is evident in the weakening, in some cases the very disappearance, of spaces of transition and delay, places where people can distinguish different conditions or phases. Such places facilitate normal passages from one state to another and are determined by the *communitas* with the manners, rituals, and rhythms typical of human needs, as Arnold Van Gennep (1909) and Victor Turner (1969) describe. The two authors argue that the notion of liminality or a border, a suspension that respects ambiguity and indeterminacy, must be introduced between detachment from the past and a new status. To reduce and sometimes to altogether cancel the rites of passage defining transitional phases is to reduce or cancel the time to ask questions and wait, that necessary time to recognise and transform oneself. Psychiatrists and architects should plan together places that allow and respect the rhythms of suffering people without using arbitrary, inconsistent, and authoritarian methods. Functional architectural solutions should not be based on simplistic, simplifying, and ambiguous demagogy because this reduces the possibility of autonomy and psychophysical regeneration, two of the main goals which safeguard and promote curing.

These places must include together public and domestic features through a continuous mixture of known and unknown elements and areas in which it is possible to help patients to recognise their old identities and foster their new ones inside the institution. This entails removing conventional spatial distances and defining new ones. In these new spatial distances, contact must be simultaneously warm and sufficiently formalised in order to respect the patients' suffering and avoid the absence of space that often characterises intimate relationships between people.

The space must be able to promote an emphatic but not invasive participation, to protect intimacy without being prescriptive or authoritarian, to discretely and flexibly guarantee all the patient's need to stay isolated whilst still allowing them to communicate with others when they wish to do so.

Sometimes we psychoanalysts are tempted to refer to a mythical and mythological internal world of a human being who is disconnected from the developmental stages that define them, that is, from their experiences and the accidents and contingencies of their personal history, from the instability of their boundaries. After a phase of idealisation of the division of the internal world, perhaps a reaction to the positivistic culture which does not consider the emotional and affective determinants in the observation of facts, we recognised that knowing and taking care of the internal world require both leaving some preclusive and eliminative competencies and assuming a curious attention and a careful cure towards the external world without cuts or breaks. For Freud (1933),[2] the internal world cannot be not only internal: the internal world also breaks into and transform the composition, partition, and boundaries of the external world in an endless osmosis. A great part of our identity is outside us, in the objects around us, the furniture and decorative objects of our rooms, in our clothes, in our paths. The skin, the surface of our body, is a sort of osmotic membrane that divides the internal from the external space. An inefficacious regulation of exchanges projects the suffering in our internal world on objects and external space in general. We can experience this space as fragmented or weird and unrecognisable. Objects can become estranged and threatening.

When they develop community spaces, architects ought to plan areas of containment and cure that deal with the distinction or lack of distinction between Self and non-Self, between chaos and order, between the differentiated and the undifferentiated. Spaces ought to address multiple and complex needs, compositions, and decompositions of the subject, constructions, and deconstructions. They ought to host those parts of our mind we still consider hostile and needing to expel, repress, ban, or order. Giving considerable attention to space that will contain mental disease, through which we can walk or go through and observe according to the criteria of a great part of the architectonic production, can widen both the sense and the senses, transform the *Unheimlich* in *Heimlich*, without comfortable cognitive heuristics, and directly connect bodily language and physical space, between the unconscious and its habitat. Such an approach bestows containment functions to living spaces that have lacked them because they have never accommodated those features of the mind that cannot be ordered without strong yet ineffective repression. They are spaces in which the need for shelter and the desire to expose oneself are in conflict. They are spaces with contradictions and conflicts that do not seek a false (because it is imposed) quiet. In fact, authentic hospitality favours the expression of the numerous Egos living there, the constitutive otherness of the Ego, everything belonging to the human being in order to then be able to accept it.

Certainly, it is mandatory to avoid automatic and ideological transpositions through which spaces that suggest disorder, instability, precariousness, or incompleteness allow mental suffering. This is in opposition to the repressive and almost deadly spatial and temporal order typical of the psychiatric hospital and many other community places. Architectonic spaces can modify human relationships and behaviour not only because they are conceived and organised with specific functions and scopes: relationships and behaviours are deeply rooted in culture, habit, and social convention. However, because they contain emotions and actions, these spaces can intervene and influence the transformative processes of a person, their vicissitudes, communications, and behaviours. This can be achieved only if they are not uniform and exclusive. These spaces can be transformed from neutrality, passivity, and logic to activity, involvement, and stimulation, to an openness to the personal needs of its inhabitants. They can provide comfort, confidence, and even a quiet comprehension and acceptance of what it is different and unfamiliar, existing between the logic of sharing and aggression, among people who can be involved or not in public spaces, open or not towards other people. Places dedicated to treating psychic suffering must be conceived and created as complete environmental units that include spaces for resting and waiting, interstitial spaces apt to intense exchanges and relationships between people. Such transitional spaces stimulate a true and genuine search for harmony between the needs of patients and their caregivers (Schinaia, 2019).

The Monasterial Path

The architecture of the monastery, a place for hospitality and human relationships, can serve as a useful reference for the design of a psychiatric community. The cell is the most private place: it is both maternal because it is intimate and containing, intended for sleeping, and paternal because it is intended for contemplating, concentrating, and studying. Through careful and balanced modalities we arrive at the cloister, where cells overlook a common court with a garden at its centre. Surrounding the garden is an arcade that connects the indoor and outdoor and functions as a space in which we can have an intimate and whispered conversation or a silent but collective meditation.

Here the threads of attention are intertwined inside and outside ourselves and move themselves between our irreducible singularity and the assorted composition of a community (Boatti, 2012). Next, we have the chapter house, a public and paternal space in which most meetings about the activities of the monastery and its community take place. This is the place for the democracy of opinions and emotions, in which leadership is expressed through listening. Here the monks not only discuss the agenda or elect the abbot, the admission to novitiate, the purchase and sale of plots of land, but also collectively deal with intimate personal questions, for example, when a brother is in an existential or religious crisis. The chapter house is the first example of effective democracy: in it the monks are free to express their opinions on the issues of the monastery. Then there is the church, with the oratory and choir, in which each monk has a bench to occupy, standing with his elbows on the armrests. Perhaps the church is the main place in which ritualised and organised oral communication takes place and in which the day ends with the compline, the final prayer of the day.

There are also corridors and the library, a place for reading and preserving books. Finally, we have the refectory, the place in which to feed the body and the soul. Exchanges are still ritualised here but less formal and constrained, thus much freer. They are a prelude to a sociality that prefigures the outside, in other words, the exit from the monastery to the open square and thus to the world. Different working activities occurring in purpose-built areas having the aspect of small shops accompany this exit (Marazzi, 2015).

I believe that we should be inspired by Franciscan cloisters: in order to contain social and individual needs in a creative way, they removed the strong normativity and rigid repetitiveness that are typical of monks' days and are established in their ancient manuals or formalised rules (*regulae*) from the monastery's spaces. This enables the flexible use of different spaces and thus of adequately expressing different languages without an *a priori* excessively formalised manner, allowing multiple adequate functional expressions and communicative possibilities.[3] Monastery life is based not only on the laws of fraternity but also on those of hospitality: the community is so well grounded that it can receive foreign and unknown elements without changing its rhythms in any way.

As Petrella (1993a) clearly points out, the aim here is to render accessible and treatable those dimensions of the mind in which the distinction between the Self and the non-Self is still uncertain or lost. This necessitates the construction of environments able to contain and receive this lack of distinction. In other words, we need specific and specialised settings. Perhaps we should create spaces able to adequately receive those imaginary constructs that have no place in the world, those ghosts we used to put in a hidden world full of the wishes, fears, hates, and needs that we find in our patients. This is a feeling of being out of place, typical of psychosis. But, of course, this is also our feeling.

We hope it can be a prelude to us recovering ourselves, reorganising our daily life and using new and different methods of communication.

Institutional Reanimation and Rehabilitation

Reflections on the places for therapy are valuable not only for all those who are ill but also for all health workers. The latter need an environment that can recognise their suffering, too, and allow a form of its elaboration, so as to avoid the activation of strong psychic defence mechanisms, difficulties in communication, and high levels of anxiety. In fact, these distortions can result in occupational burnout and institutionalisation and, as a consequence, create obstacles to efficiency in the entire health system.

The restoration and preservation of the Nativity scene and its positioning in an adequate structure which can give value to its beauty and originality should lead to the recognition of the history of psychiatric care services and the stories of the people who were so unlucky to live and die in a psychiatric hospital. This holds true not only for today's health care workers and public but also for future generations.

This book proposes to look at the Nativity scene in Cogoleto from a psychoanalytic point of view.

It is a reflection on the risks involved when we propose the old psychiatric institutionalisation in new forms. Although psychiatric hospitals no longer exist in Italy, there is a tendency to not recognise the psychological needs of people who suffer by trying to reduce mental disorders only at the biological level. To do so is to envision the psychiatric hospital in modern, sophisticated, and thus mystifying ways. As Eugenio Gaburri (1994) stresses, the Basaglia Law buried the institution. But the institution could rise like a phoenix from the ashes and prevent the physician-patient relationship that can get at the essence of mental anguish in a way no psychotropic drug can.

We must oppose scientific practices and ideologies based on biologistic claims that lead to pharmacological therapy devoid of any relational intention or ability to consider patients' existential and emotional needs, inner worlds, and affective vicissitudes. We are in the midst of the revival of a descriptive psychiatry based on highly defensive diagnostic classifications of mental disorders. They aim to classify, distinguish, and separate, and they arrogantly devaluate the medical classification of symptoms in order to associate the correct psychotropic drug.

Similarly, the uncritical acceptance of certain forms of cognitive-behavioural therapy is dangerous. By sidestepping the deepest fears, incomprehensible silences, and seemingly meaningless words, it allows healers to distance themselves from that difficult but irreplaceable emotional and empathic contact with suffering women and men.

The institutional reanimation that, as a psychoanalyst, I tried to effect along with my therapeutic team was the first attempt to directly deal with chronicity. It was an anti-entropic effort, in opposition to the tendency towards stasis, stillness, and non-differentiation. We proposed care and cures based on movement, rhythm, space, and time, all elements that the experience of life in a psychiatric hospital had inevitably eliminated.

> *"Giving a name to the patients, reconstructing, or constructing together a possible story, helping them to keep pace with a non-deadly daily routine had been complex operations that had required a deep knowledge of psychoanalysis and group therapy for avoiding behaviourism and a form of simplistic pedagogy."* (Schinaia, 1998b, p. 105)

Reanimation can be fully performed only if the psychoanalyst is able to guarantee the symbolic level of all the rehabilitative operations and provide a narrative framework for them.

A behaviouristic-pedagogical approach considers the patient as a person who needs previously lacking possibilities and ways to learn how to perform certain functions (professional, artistic, manual, etc.) that the chronicity of their mental disease blocked. This approach does not consider that the insistence on the patient's productive, socialising, and practical aspects can promote their splits if it is not accompanied by a process of psychical working through and thus of mental growth. In other words, this approach can reinforce a False Self adapted to the context but distinct from the patient's dramatic and afflicted (or empty) inner world. Because lack of cohesion or unity of Selves is one of the most common problems for these patients, this aspect must be at the centre of their therapies, not their practical or behavioural performances (Correale, 1991).

The aim of rehabilitation is to help the patient to activate an internal creative process, not to fill a blank mental space or solve a problem (Hochmann, 1992). It follows that rehabilitation should re-activate desire and creativity and oppose those destructive tendencies that had almost always characterised the patients' development, making it difficult or highly disharmonious (Petrella, 1993b).

The planning, creation, and conservation of the Nativity scene in Cogoleto served the function of reanimating a comatose institutional life. By giving voice not only to the patients' pain and fear but also to their desire and hope, it was a form of symbolic re-appropriation. Its narrative and representational capacity teemed with therapeutic potential by allowing the recovery of frozen, barren, unknown, or unrecognised parts of the Self and the discovery and experience of previously unimaginable propulsive movement and creativity.

Notes

1 The term "interstice" comes from the Latin *interstitium* and means "to stay between," in other words, to be in an undefined situation that is anomic in certain aspects or, at least, that does not follow a set of formal rules of order and organisation. Cianconi (2013) argues that the interstice is not necessarily a defined place that remains stable over time, functional, or balanced.

2 Freud (1933) writes, "internal foreign *territory—just as reality (if you will forgive the unusual expression)* is external foreign territory" (p. 140). He distinguishes internal foreign territory from the external world that he calls reality or external foreign territory.
3 In the settlements of the Order of Preachers and the Mendicant Orders, next to the places where the communities lived and which were closed to outsiders (the so-called *caesurae*), there was a new radical conception of the space of the church, a place entirely open access to the believer (Marazzi, 2015).

Foreword by Fausto Petrella[1]

This book by Cosimo Schinaia is a peculiar literary work, anomalous and different, like the Nativity scene that inspired it. It must be considered as a *sui generis* work composed of many different parts and sources. Its unique character is one of the strengths of the work and the source of its lively originality. This aspect can benefit from an introductive reflection and inform the reader. Thus, I propose a simple introduction to the book and not an attempt to situate it in a well-defined literary genre.

When I wrote this introduction, per the request of the author—a psychoanalyst, psychiatrist, former loyal student of Dario De Martis and mine in Pavia, and then talented director of Cogoleto Psychiatric Hospital—my mind returned to my personal experiences in the psychiatric hospital. These experiences are still living and breathing even for those like me, who were so lucky as to not be fully involved in them quite soon (for me just before 1978). Those who experienced the psychiatric hospital (as I did for a decade, more or less) can find many similarities with life in a lager or prison. Many doctors, nurses, and patients rightly made this parallel. Those who had this experience, no matter if psychiatrists or nurses, were strongly marked in different ways. Today the problem is how to give testimony about this reality that appears very far in time, especially for young people, but that it is actually very near and whose traces persist. All psychiatrists know that only the death of those who shared this experience will erase the traces that must not be forgotten or denied. I do not write these words with pessimism. But I cannot deny them. A survivor's testimony is certainly moving but, most of all, unwelcome by almost all, no matter if they are young and do not want to know or old hospital workers who do not want to remember. I think (it is more a feeling than a real thought) that nostalgia cannot mitigate the disturbing memory of images, people, and situations experienced in a psychiatric hospital. In my case, I was in Cagliari and Voghera psychiatric hospitals, not in that of Genoa, but things were the same. The reminiscent and nostalgic tones, often characterised by lyrical accents and pathetic and idealising identifications, can sometimes be found in the words of physicians who witnessed these situations and now love to write about them. These physicians were constantly in touch with the reality of the psychiatric hospital and believed themselves able to distil precious human essences from the horror they witnessed. But such essences can be found everywhere, even in the most degraded contexts. I do not like the psychiatrists-writers who exhibit these essences in their writings: they remind me of the old category of "false consciousness." The writing is certainly the paradigmatic mean through which memory becomes a document, but it always seemed to me insufficient and highly mystifying in providing truly adequate descriptions of the reality of the psychiatric hospital. I have always felt that every narrative "fiction," however sensitive and committed, cannot represent the pathos of direct experience, the vertigo of disorientation, or the miserable horror of the teeming and estranged humanity living in the medical structures of mental illness.

It is difficult to clearly represent an extreme experience such as that of alienation, an overused word. I'm also dissatisfied with poetry and its immense expressive possibilities as well as with cinematic representations of mental disease in psychiatric institutions. There are of course some exceptions and perhaps I can appear too harsh and uncompromising. However, it is a matter of fact that a paradigmatic book similar to *Survival in Auschwitz* by Primo Levi (1947) but about life in a psychiatric institution still does not exist. It should be a mix between the estranged perspective of a valuable and slightly mad anthropologist and the ardour of Dostoevsky's *Notes from the Underground* (1864) combined with Carlo Emilio Gadda's lucid hyperaesthesia for the grotesque and disharmonic plurality of voices of the world represented in *That Awful Mess on Via Merulana* (1957).

It is mandatory for those who write about the psychiatric hospital and represent its contrasts and aporias to propose a pastiche or something messy, an "awful mess" in Gadda's terms, in order to approach their object of inquiry, putting together the shocking truth of a lived experience with the truth of writing, no matter if scientific or artistic.

Cosimo Schinaia is not only a passionate and indignant witness: he is also an active supporter of the project of overcoming the psychiatric hospitals. He produced a harsh patchwork: because of my personal knowledge of the author, I can assure that he could not have softened the contents of his book in an impressionistic manner. This work of his is much more than a testimony of a past and present clinical, welfare, and human reality: it is also a document reporting a historical transformation and criticism of the medical and social practice of psychiatric violence.

Further, it presents not only important ethical and humanitarian considerations but also technical ones. Finally, it has a precise systematicity, and thus it is also both a sort of manual and a small museum of horrors. Schinaia uses the Cogoleto Nativity scene, an oxymoronic, tender, and controversial work of art, as a plot or map with all its indications and fundamental stations. This Nativity is the basic structure of the whole discourse, so that the book finds in the Nativity its illustration, its pretext, and even what must receive an answer. This devoted and popular theatre, sometimes rustic and poor, sometimes childish and baroque, offers to both children and adults the naive and captivating show of the nativity of Jesus and the coming of the child God, with his family, in the human world.

In this artwork, the Christian mystery of the incarnation of God is reduced to a human size and set in a landscape and habit that represents the point of strength of the mimetic narrative mode. Here we can find many elements of rural and peasant life, the different jobs and trades, the figurines fixed in the various activities in the countryside, woods, villages, and hills. The spectator can observe all both in general, from a panoramic perspective, and particular, in its details. There are also graceful self-propeled Nativity scenes which represent the child God and the world as well-ordered and providentially organised. This indicates that the Child is postulated to be surrounded by a firm, solid, and well-defined natural and social world. This is an unreliable picture because it is evident to all that the infant's construction and introduction in the limited reality of society and culture is long and difficult. But in the Nativity scene God and the Child are the same, as the amazing and mythical intuition of Christianism postulates, and everything goes very well, at least in the beginning. Can we imagine an updated version of the Nativity scene, perhaps more modern and current? Certainly, someone just did it, for example, by changing the traditional rural landscape with a modern and urban setting, with cars, miniature trains, rockets, armed soldiers, and the Three Wise Men riding motorcycles.

Renaissance painters made great use of such anachronisms and received public acclaim and approval. Some theatre, film, or opera directors do the same today when, not always happily, they offer up mythological divinities and historical characters in modern clothes or equip the conquering Romans with the most recent weapons, etc. We all know that these updates are seldom artistically sound but, when they work, they enhance and help us to better understand the deep meaning of the work of Sophocles, Shakespeare, or Handel. There has certainly been someone in the theatre who set their play in the unstable place *par excellence*, the psychiatric hospital. I think of Jerzy Grotowski, the inventor of the "poor theatre," who organised his theatrical action with some scenes typical of the psychiatric hospital and set them very close to the audience. This stripped the audience of the reassuring comfort of the stage and replaced it with the patient's position.

But I think that no one had ever thought to set the Holy Family of the Nativity scene in a psychiatric hospital, substituting the countryside landscape with the threatening structure of the hospital, with its cells, isolation and medical rooms, room for the electroshock, etc. In this

Nativity scene, doctors, nurses, and patients, with all their factions and parts, replace shepherds, peasants, and artisans. Every Christmas, in many Italian psychiatric wards, as well as in many other medical settings, nurses set up Christmas trees and Nativity scenes, as parents do with their children in their homes. There is nothing strange about this: was not the psychiatric ward the home of many long-term patients? Those poor Christmas arrangements and decorations recall this neatly and mercilessly, even though they are acts of sympathy and solidarity.

But the Nativity scene of Cogoleto is something different and clearly original. It had been conceived and created by patients and nurses, as well as a professional artist. It must be preserved and maintained, not dismantled after the celebration ends. At the anthropologically level, this scene can be considered as the expression of a culture and art in strong opposition to those of the psychiatric institution, a non-place with no gods or art, without a true communicative link to that hegemonic culture of which the Nativity scene itself is a lovely symbol.

The Nativity scene of Cogoleto breaks this distinction and contraposition and constitutes a sort of ceremony of the opposites; that is, in a provocative manner, it connects the *Spaltung* of a founding cultural paranoia that separates and creates dualism between value and disvalue, sane and insane, world and non-world. The Nativity scene is a unifying expression and representation. Perhaps Christ stopped at Cogoleto, as he did at Eboli, as reported by Carlo Levi (1945). This unifying act could be the starting gesture of a new impossible culture, in which the institution in its totality bursts into the outside and becomes part of the world, not its secret and hidden counterpart. This ceremony of the opposites that cannot coexist is almost unconceivable, except in an artistic discourse: indeed, today's post-psychiatric institutional rehabilitative practices actually propose it.

At the artistic level, this ceremony is something sublime, where at the social level it can be a symbol of evangelisation of the barbarian or a carnivalesque attack on the holy. But, above all, there is a clear fact: the oneiric connection between the holy and some specific secular features is thought-provoking; that is, it forces the spectator to critique and reflect. This is the same reflection that permitted the creation of such a ceremony of the opposites: it is not clear if it desecrates or mocks, but it is certainly an efficacious general social criticism. The world of each one of us is an unacknowledged collective psychiatric hospital. The presence of Genoa in the landscape should exclude this interpretation and give the spectator a sort of reassurance.

Around the artwork and the idea of a psychiatric Nativity scene, Schinaia wrote both an important anti-manual of psychiatry and the tale of a clinical reality, *forma mentis*, and system of life: that of the institutional psychiatry, with an attempt to ideologically and practically transcend it.

He wrote this book to remind us of the institutionalisation of violence in psychiatry and denounce one more time, but in an original form, both the possibility that science can do something against the defenceless madness and the deep reasons why this happened in the history of modern medicine and could happen in the future, perhaps in different and unexpected ways.

Note

1 Fausto Petrella (1938–2020) was a psychiatrist, psychoanalyst, head of the psychiatric clinic of the Faculty of Medicine at the University of Pavia, and president of the Italian Psychoanalytic Society.

Introduction to the Italian Edition

From the point of view of those visiting the Nativity scene in Cogoleto, the representation of the psychiatric hospital follows the principle that there must be a full correspondence between reality and its artistic transfiguration. Thus, the series of scenes of the Nativity cannot be considered arbitrary or invented. Rather, they precisely reproduce the spatial organisation and the functional and topological distribution of all the different parts of the hospital. Further, the play of the light and perspective allows emotional access to that atmosphere of abandon and timelessness typical of life inside the institution. Immediately beyond the gate were the buildings housing the physicians' rooms, administrative offices, library, and apartments of those physicians who lived on site. People lived very close to the exit and could thus escape to the outside world in critical moments. This outside guaranteed the identity of providers of care and cures (the "normal" people) as opposed to the patients (the "crazy" people). The area immediately beyond the gate was far from the in-patient pavilions, places of sadistic segregation from which even the physicians tried to keep away as much as possible.

The patient pavilions were dispersed in a wide area, closed and inaccessible. Each contained small rooms in which agitated people or those who troubled the inhuman institutional order were segregated, an anonymous living room in which every form of socialisation and communication was impossible and a so-called square, a court that was the extension of the living room, an external space that was rigorously enclosed. Each ward also had a room for electroconvulsive therapy, a space full of pain and mystery, usually placed near the medical room, at the centre of the pavilion as a sort of memento or menace for the patients, as if the scared faces and screams of pain could have prevented the disturbance of institutional order.

The paediatric ward and the school near it were separated from other pavilions, preventing any contact with adults and the risk that they could assault the children. Like the other parts of the hospital, they had the same characteristics of abandonment and relational isolation.

Past the buildings lay a wide expanse of many fields with olive and fruit trees, a pigpen, some poultry, and cows. Here were also a carpentry shop, a laundry, a mechanical workshop, and some other workshops.

The series of scenes of the Nativity reflect the idea at the basis of Cogoleto Psychiatric Hospital architecturally and functionally. Cogoleto was different from most other psychiatric hospitals because its architecture was not based on a phalanstery. There was neither a central part from which a series of radiating wings departed (and thus less staff were needed to control all the movement of patients from the centre) nor concentric circles (in which the wards were infernal circles that became more terrifying as they went from the periphery to the centre, where the agitated people were kept).

The gate and medical rooms on one side and the fields on the other were the borders of the disseminated pavilion village. These borders were not so neat as in other institutions; they were disguised and embellished with high hedges and impassable. Near the hedges was Cogoleto's cemetery, neatly divided into one part for Cogoleto's residents, that the patients could not access, and another part for the patients, a sadly egalitarian area, in which all the anonymous crosses were identical, distinguished only by a number that the passage of time first faded and then erased.

The most important variants that the amateur artists (no matter if patient, nurse, staff, or physician) conceded themselves during the creation of the Nativity scene can be found in the Nativity itself at the beginning of the artwork. It is a full-size Nativity reminiscent of the deep emotional-affective meaning that the birth and belonging to a group hold for these patients. At the end of the artwork, is a breathtaking panorama of Genoa, from its harbour to its hills, a city characterised by the daring colours of the facades of its buildings. I think that for the patients these colours represented the hope of returning to their place of origin, a hope they almost lost.

In the traditional Nativity the theme of the journey scene is generally conceived as a linear pathway towards a goal: the cave, the location of that mysterious meeting between the human and the divine, between our finitude and the promise of our redemption (Riolfo Marengo, 1996). Instead the journey of the Cogoleto Nativity scene starts from the Nativity itself and meanders in the psychiatric hospital's labyrinth, through its deepest, darkest, and smelliest interiors, to unveil the horrors, to deal with its subtle fascination. The route is characterised by a series of intermediate stations representing the strenuous attempts to change, the weak initial needs to open up and finally to reach the desired sunny city, the open and breezy spaces of existence which repeats itself day after day, simultaneously the same and different.

This city contains all the hopes of emancipation and socialisation in which it is possible to live with other people not only without repressing the differences at the sociological level but also without rigidly and inhumanly separating.

The construction of the narrative itinerary aimed to respect the real set of the Nativity and its scenes and thus the original itinerary inside Cogoleto Psychiatric Hospital. This itinerary also aspired towards the possible light at the end of a painful and fearsome pathway, a promise to fulfil the need for freedom and maintain an expressed or apparently not expressed hope.

Every scene has a chapter, a small and autonomous monograph describing the historical, anthropological, and psychoanalytical features connected to the artistic representation. Thus, the scenes of Nativity are not still images of the past; rather, they transmit the sensation of a movement, an evolution, a future project. Of course, in order to avoid that this volume becomes a mere catalogue of an exhibition from a museum of horrors, a certain discontinuity (that sometimes is nothing but arbitrariness) is chosen and must be accepted in the presentation of the scenes. This book can be a lively tool for learning the history of the psychiatric hospital and comparing options, ideas, and projects in the controversy in contemporary psychiatry regarding the different scientific hypotheses for tending to or curing mental illness without choosing institutionalisation as a solution.

After an outline of the history of the asylum at Cogoleto (Chapter 1), from its origins to today, a description of the current plans for what to do with the former psychiatric hospital (Chapter 2) and a brief history of the work of art created there, its design and construction (Chapter 3), I describe the most significant scenes of the artwork. The asylum's representation of the nativity (Chapter 4) goes from the illustration of the anthropological features of the birth of Christ to the psychoanalytic hypotheses about its experience and memory. It shows the great need for maternity, paternity, family warmth that life inside the psychiatric hospital too often erases. The inexorably closed gate, the small isolation rooms for the agitated, the sitting room of the pavilion (Chapter 5), and the square (Chapter 6) represent the segregation, incommunicability, and radical elimination of the spatial and temporal dimensions. Perhaps the medical room (Chapter 7) is the symbol of the coarse measures some caretakers adopted to defend themselves against mental suffering. In fact, the white coats were necessary not only so that the doctors could identify one another but, more importantly, so they could differentiate themselves from the patients—and thus avoid the risk of discovering that their identity was frail and artificial. The protagonist of Chekhov's novella *Ward No. 6* (1892) is a psychiatrist who makes the mistake of excessively identifying with a paranoid patient and ends up locked up in an asylum. The electroshock room (Chapter 8) is where the caretakers' defences become more sophisticated. Here is where they exercise a technique abolishing every contact with the Other, who in turn becomes victim of arbitrary acts and abuses of power. Here also is where we can reflect on the historical roots of a therapeutic tool still in use and, as we will see, still justified at least as an extreme measure, for example, for those forms of depression that do not respond to any form of pharmacotherapy or psychotherapy, in which there is a high chance of suicide. The scenes of the paediatric ward and school (Chapter 9) underscore the lack of attention that society pays children, especially those with a severe psychophysical handicap, the delays in assistance and, more in general, the absence of a culture that favours giving help to the family of the child with mental disease over reverting to institutionalisation. The subject of work (Chapter 10) sees institutional ergotherapy (with illiberality and exploitation as its ideological roots) give way to psychosocial rehabilitation with the construction of cooperatives, with work activities that have a dimension that is both therapeutic and social. The cemetery (Chapter 11) is neatly divided in two sections, one for the "normal," the other for the "crazy," with the corpses of the latter transported in the cover of night, so as not to disturb the daily relationships outside the psychiatric hospital and cause a scandal. We feel the force of the prejudice, the intensity of the fear of becoming infected that mental disease provokes.

The description of the town of Cogoleto and Genoa la Superba (the proud one), the beautiful, big, and distant city, points towards the future, to ambitious and rich rehabilitative and therapeutic projects that can transcend the idea of the psychiatric institute. The starting point for these projects must be the enrichment of the emotional fabric at the basis of every therapeutic relationship. They must be tailored to the individual, not one size fits all, so as to avoid dangerous and ideological solutions, sociological rationalisations for not facing the deep fears that the long-term patient communicates and instills in the caretaker along with a sense of aridity, impotence, and failure.

The former patients of Cogoleto Psychiatric Hospital have the right to be compensated with a dignified future. Their nativity shows us this right.

1 Cogoleto Psychiatric Hospital

The constitution of psychiatry as an autonomous and institutionalised science in Italy can be easily traced back to the birth of the unitary state, thus starting from the half of the 19th century. This period lasted a little more than 60 years. It ended at the beginning of the First World War precisely after the enactment of the Giolitti Law on Psychiatric Hospitals (1904–1909). This law was the result of intense efforts by Italian psychiatrists.

In 1904, when the law was passed, the relationship between civil society and the psychiatric institution was definitively established without any mediation in terms of division or exclusion, absent the articulated and fruitful conflict that characterised the debate among Italian psychiatrists until that moment. This debate was between the immobilism typical of the psychiatric hospital *per se* and the big emancipatory demands, the enthusiastic explorations of anthropological and philosophical realms, and the reduction of the infinite possibilities of human existence to a few nosographic formulas and classifications that could be used daily in an administrative and bureaucratic manner.

The Giolitti Law clearly defined the organisation of psychiatric hospitals and its relationship with public administration and criminal justice. Further, it provided for indefinite control over alienated people, a control going far beyond the experience in the psychiatric hospital. In fact, article 66 of this law established the so-called experimental dismissal, a sort of indefinite conditional release that the psychiatric system could revoked at will. The registration of internment in a psychiatric hospital in the criminal record created an irrevocable link with the justice system and provided a tool for the systematic control of future generations (Giacanelli, 1980).

The asylum became the physical and relational space, the *topos*, of the cure of mental disease, the sum of every therapeutical path defined by the new psychiatric science (Canosa, 1979). But history told us that asylums were places in which the reality of human and social marginality and disintegration was suspended. The waste of capitalistic society was all stuffed in real human storages into which the alienated person

DOI: 10.4324/9781003381723-1

irremediably lost any hope to reconnect the broken links with external reality (De Bernardi et al., 1980).

The social framework from which Italian psychiatry emerged in those years was characterised by the drama of misery, chronic under-feeding, and degradation of human and hygienic conditions of large segments of population (from Northern farmers to Southern labourers) (Giacanelli, 1975).

Around the middle of the 19th century, reducing the number of patients in the building on via Galata in Genoa became an urgent necessity. Until then, the building was the only official psychiatric hospital in Liguria. It housed far more than the 400 "maniacs" for which it was designed.

The asylum on via Galata was a sort of monument to custody. It was not only inadequate due to its capacity and phalansterial structure but also according to the most modern scientific principles. It was situated in a central urban area, which the still-young Italian positivistic psychiatry considered dangerous for both the patients and neighbourhood inhabitants (Babini et al., 1982).

The 8th Congress of Italian Scientists, held in Genoa in 1845, mandated that future buildings such as that on via Galata could not be too large and had to always be situated outside the city so that patients could farm the land (Carpaneto, 1953). Thus, finding a large space outside the city—a salubrious area with abundance of water in which to establish fields that patients could cultivate—was mandatory.

To create those living conditions adequate for a high number of chronic patients, for whom there was neither hope nor chance of social reintegration, a psychiatric hospital with a complex and articulated structure was necessary.

Francesco Azzurri (1877), an architect who extensively studied the structures of psychiatric hospitals, stressed the need to go beyond symmetric and monumental forms such as those of the building on via Galata, with its hospital-like construction evoking a place of confinement. He intended to design a place in which peace, order and community life were the values of the curing project under the guidance of medical science. The result was so-called scattered village system, with multiple buildings (pavilions) forming a small village whose aim was to be a colony for the insane. In other words, the aim of this system was to create an autonomous, self-sufficient micro-community according to the parameters of an ideal society of normal people (De Peri, 1984).

In the annual balance sheet of 1924, the head of the Cogoleto Psychiatric Hospital wrote that the pavilions were variously scattered and equally spaced, arranged all along wide tree-lined avenues, giving the unexpected impression of wandering around an elegant village. This spared the new hospital of the usual repulsive aspect of such buildings and made it appear different from the customary severe and prison-like institutions.

The attempt to open and enlarge the spatial context in which to put the patients could appear on the one hand as a partial alternative and an implicit condemnation of the most segregating aspects of the psychiatric hospital and on the other as something functional to both the ideology of work and the alleged necessity to limit the use of psychiatric hospitalisation (De Bernardi et al., 1980).

The public administration of the Province of Genoa received various proposals for land, former convents, and properties. One interesting proposal came from Cogoleto: 100 hectares described as propitious and not expensive.

The report of the commission in charge of evaluating the opportunities for the construction of a psychiatric hospital in Cogoleto pointed out that the place was appropriate according to the principles of the modern technology of building psychiatric hospitals. It appeared to be perfect for the construction of an asylum as a scattered village, without covered hallways, like those in Meerenberg in Holland or Mendrisio in Switzerland. What's more, the land was 160–180 metres above sea level, exposed at midday, well defended from the North wind by a 250-metre high buttress, surrounded by woods, and made cheerful by views of the Apennines and the Ligurian sea.

There was one problem: it was too far from the city of Genoa and very difficult for the patients' relatives to reach. In 1889, the government authority temporarily stopped the project because of the considerations of many Italian psychiatrists and the pressure from many academics in Genoa. Only in 1895 could Genoa have a new asylum in the district of Quarto. But in no time it could not handle the high number of admissions.

In April 1909 some physicians—horrified that patients were jumbled and confused, with nary a comfort, condemned to physical and mental deterioration—demanded that provincial authorities make a formal inquiry into the functioning of psychiatric hospitals. They argued that they did not want to be accomplices to such an offence against the most basic principles of civilisation and human mercy.

The problem returned after 18 years, when the asylum of via Galata was set to be demolished and the Psychiatric Hospital of Quarto, opened in 1895, was declared excessively full.

The never-ending story of, first, the project for Cogoleto and, then, during the first years of the past century, its construction, is a paradigmatic example of the various contradictory interests among the different institutions having to manage the mentally ill (Molinari A., 1994). The demolition of the building on via Galata increased the value of the surrounding areas, which were sold, with the proceeds going towards the construction of a public hospital in the neighbourhood of San Martino. The psychiatric hospital was moved out of the city centre mainly for financial reasons.

In 1908, the project of the Psychiatric Hospital of Cogoleto was approved. The border of the province of Genoa was moved to facilitate its construction and include the district of Cogoleto and the new hospital (Masini, 1908).

The asylum was structured in pavilions and covered 100 hectares. It was the largest in Liguria and, according to the project, could hold 2,400 patients. It opened in 1912. Ten pavilions were ready. Three were added later that year; three more in 1921–1922; and the final three in 1933. Despite the plans for a specific use of the various pavilions, the quantity of requests brought to occupy the pavilions as they were set up. This meant to delay the decision of a more logical arrangement of the departments.

In 1912 the number of patients in the Quarto and Cogoleto hospitals was 2,300. Two years later, there were 900 in Cogoleto alone. The overcrowding persisted. Two years after Cogoleto opened, it had to send some patients to asylums in other parts of Italy. As many psychiatrists had predicted 50 years before, Cogoleto could accommodate only a small number of the ill, and it was soon transformed into a depository of lunatics (Molinari A., 1994).

The expansion of Cogoleto and the construction of new pavilions in Quarto in the years between the two World Wars did not solve the problem of overcrowding. In fact, admissions in Genoa were constantly higher compared to the national average, at least until the 1930s.

By 1924, there were 2,200 patients at Cogoleto. Because it was considered a branch of the central quarter, it was subordinated to its sister facility in Quarto starting in 1928. If it were not possible to send all the patients out of the city centre, it was possible to send some of them to Cogoleto. The doctors at Quarto chose the most derelict patients, the ones considered less tolerable and more disturbing: children affected by cerebropathy, people with cognitive deficits, those with tuberculosis.

This is a story of losers: women, men, and children unable to withstand the physical and psychical weight of misery and exploitation. Progress meant a continuous loss of their mental faculties, a complete disappearance of their Selves. Imbeciles, cretins, pellagrous, alcoholic, goitred, demented, and hysterical patients were only the annoying human waste of progress: a form of degeneration that psychiatrists and the institute must cure and rehabilitate for civil cohabitation, but in reality remove, render inoffensive and socially non-existing (De Bernardi et al., 1980).

A multitude of patients could be indiscriminately concentrated far beyond the limits of environmental space and hygienic concerns. This is evident in the annual budget report of 1925, in which the head of the asylum praised its location and invisibility to those who searched for it in the village of Cogoleto.

In the first years of the institute, the nursing staff were composed of single mothers, war widows, and strong men at least 1.64 metres tall.

All had only to be able to read and write. They generally came from the poorest regions of Italy or at best from the city of Genoa: the locals despised the jobs inside the asylum. Later, working in the institute became a sort of familiar heritage to be handed down from generation to generation among the inhabitants of Cogoleto and its surrounding villages.

The physicians lived in a sort of garrison atmosphere, in buildings around or inside the structure; the nurses worked 12-hour shifts and slept in special dormitories in the pavilions, sometimes locked in, just like the patients.

As Tanzi (1905) points out, in the citadel inhabited by the hopeless, psychiatrists could only feel condemned to intellectual degradation. Their only task was disciplinary surveillance. It is not a case that as time went by the prestige of the physicians working in the asylum greatly declined. This happened also at the juridical and salary level: they were considered inferior to their colleagues working in the hospital (Scarcella et al., 1980).

Maura and Pisseri (1991) write that we can lock up the madman with no remorse if we lock up with him one of our delegates, who has a place in our imagination, like Christ *qui tollis peccata mundi* ("who takes away the sins from the world"). Should the madman deal with an impossible task and fall into distrust, inertia, and cynicism, with the inevitable omnipotent-manic implications, no one beyond the walls of the institute will know; or, if it becomes known and public, every fault will fall on him and the collective good conscience will be retained.

Culturally and geographically isolated, the asylum in Cogoleto soon developed an autonomous economy comparable to the court model of a medieval castle (Bosazzi and Venezia, 1986), or, Calvino's (1972, p. 69) words, it became *a city made only of exceptions, exclusions, incongruities, and contradictions.*

According to regulations, the hospital was considered as specialising in experimenting and rationally and widely employing the most evolved and advanced systems of the psychiatric technique and occupational therapy of mental disease. The aim was to re-educate the mental invalids and recover their attitudes and productive possibilities, thus getting the highest and most worthwhile results from helping the incurable.

An agricultural colony with cattle, pigs, and poultry farms was built, as were a bakery, pasta factory, laundry, printing press, and carpentry and ironwork workshops. Despite working at full speed and producing goods, the patient workers were not adequately paid because occupational therapy was considered a moral rather than a rehabilitative cure. The most brutal acts of segregation and exploitation went hand in hand with humanitarian and therapeutic motivations. The products were mainly consumed inside the hospital, in a self-sufficient circuit.

There was also an operating room mainly for performing lobotomies but sometimes used for general surgery. This was done to avoid transferring the mentally ill to the public hospital: the psychiatrists also cured internal pathologies, preventing every contact with the hospital doctors. Psychiatric illness put all other pathologies in the background: medical autarky was the answer to prejudice and stigma. Psychiatric symptoms were overestimated; somatic symptoms, the main cause of the high mortality rate in the psychiatric hospital, were underestimated.

In addition to the kitchen, cellars, pantries, refectory, church, theatre, anatomical museum, and mortuary, a school for hospitalised children was built. Electricity was produced autonomously, so the asylum assumed the features of a closed world.

The architectural principle according to which the spaces were designed was that of "no restraint": comfortable streets surrounded the pavilions; hedges and plants masked the net or wall closures in those points considered indispensable; the closure of the factory simply consisted of a metal net supported by iron uprights.

The pavilions were attractively painted. Each could house about 53 inmates. Over the years, the structure and agricultural colony became larger and consisted of nine employees and 30 patients who received a modest symbolic payment in recognition of work done and, the most important privilege of all, a glass of wine at each meal.

After every ambition for care through work was overcome, the agricultural colony could resume an important function. It was assumed that the work taking place in open air, fields, or airy rooms could act on chronic patients as a coefficient of hygiene and calm. It was interpreted as a tool able to reduce their mortality, without being considered a specific treatment tool in and of itself (Tanzi, 1905).

By the second half of the 1960s these practices began to be regarded as a form of deceptive humanisation on the part of an anti-human institution that was strengthened through this transformation of the patient into subordinate worker. In other words, the curative and therapeutic intention was revealed to have been hiding exploitation.

Unfortunately, these activities were not replaced by forms of jobs more respectful of human dignity. Only today can we find cooperative projects restoring the immense rural estate that was completely abandoned and limiting inactivity, regressive laziness, and lack of interest typical of the institutional days.

Although throughout the years labels and denominations changed— for example, from "asylum" to "psychiatric hospital," from "demented, maniac, alienated" to "mentally ill," etc.—madness, misery, alienation, and abandon tragically remained the same. The immutability could be seen in the pictures of the patients pasted on the title page of the yellowed and wrinkled medical records (Schinaia et al., 1992).

The main feature of the hospitalised was their anonymity: personal and identifying aspects were not considered. This solidified a general state of regression, passivity, impermeability to interpersonal relationships, and closure to contact with the external world. Medical records were poor when it came to information about patients' lives but rich with vacuous nosographic classifications. These classifications could not tell anything about personal events: they were but pseudo-scientific aberrations that revealed the nonsense of institutional practice. They look like a prison file and are organised to detect the most detailed, objective, and anthropometric signs of the stigmata of degeneration (Schinaia and Soldi, 1985).

On the title page of the medical records was the picture of the convict-patient: it was taken at the entrance of the institution, at the moment in which the facial expressions were not modified by the strong and chronic use of institutional therapies. The picture should assume the meaning of a bureaucratic identification in a situation of overcrowding with a very infrequent relationship between doctors and patients and also make a scientific diagnosis of social danger through the use of measurable bodily gestures. As a consequence, the highest ideological prejudice was linked with the highest demand of objectivity and sought a *more geometrico* (in a geometrical method) demonstration (Bollati, 1979).

The coming to power of the Fascist regime prevented Italian psychiatry to gain an autonomous scientific status by overcoming the cultural isolation from the other medical sciences. Italian psychiatry was also late in its development in comparison to the rest of Europe. As with every totalitarian regime, the Fascist regime increased this isolation because of its obsessive preoccupation towards order (De Martis, 1987). More than ever, the public perceived psychiatric institutes as isolated and dangerous.

The autarkic ambitions, xenophobic drives, and anti-Semitic prejudices long prevented access to disciplines such as the German phenomenology and Freudian psychoanalysis. Italian psychiatry was forced to form its foundations on a form of neurologism without perspectives and an idealism devoid of social and historical determinants. This furthered the distance from moral and humanitarian reasons which were at the basis of the construction of the asylum. A shortsighted scientistic positivism was favoured: it became the justification of the most aberrant and unjustified repressive practices. During the long scientific slumber of the Fascist regime, Italian psychiatry found its mediocre place. In fact, Italian psychiatry and its long institutional history followed the fate of a repressed and regimented society, from which it began to recover after the Second World War (Giacanelli, 1975).

From the end of the 19th century until the end of the Second World War, a long silence fell over the asylums. These places were silent years for millions of individuals who stayed inside those walls, millions of non-lives without voices and echoes (De Frémenville, 1977).

Since the First World War, Italian psychiatry had been engaged in a continuous effort to rehabilitate patients in order to employ them in the defence of the aims of the country. Many phrenasthenics, pure imbeciles, and epileptics were employed in the infrastructures at the front of the war or behind the scenes. In the meantime, Cesare Lombroso developed hypotheses about the usefulness of reckless psychopaths and criminals in the assaults occurring during warfare (Editorship "Psychiatry Notebooks"—"Quaderni di Psichiatria", 1917).

The same happened during the Second World War. The patient workforce was exploited to the maximum. The experience of the Nazi concentration camps, in some ways comparable to that of the asylums, and the fight for liberation involved thousands and thousands of men, women, and children but was not a lesson for the new democratic administrations. Physicians and nurses who fought the Fascist violence found themselves needing to manage the violence of the lagers-asylums and to work as jailers and guardians without feeling any contradiction.

The possibility to radically transform Italian laws or legislation on the psychiatric institution could be found in the new Constitution of the republic, which in 1948 proposed a series of rights completely incompatible with the psychiatric regime. Unfortunately, it was largely a missed opportunity. The 1904 law remained, even when the Italian Constitutional Court moved to remove the legislative system (Scarcella et al., 1980).

The number of hospitalised people continued to increase. In 1955 the hospitals of Quarto and Cogoleto held 3,304 people; a decade later, 3,614. So, too, expenses for psychiatric care constantly increased, without a better quality in services, as denounced in the *Libro Bianco sui Manicomi Genovesi* (the white book on the psychiatric hospitals of Genoa) written by the Sindacati Confederali (confederate unions) (1974).

Psychiatric care started to be criticised at the political level. Its methods, aims, and, more generally, scientific status were strongly attacked. Different experiences, debates, and workshops translated in the Mariotti Law (1968) that, in theory, wanted to put the care and services of psychiatric hospitals at the same level as those of public hospitals. The Mariotti Law proposed two innovations: the possibility of voluntary hospitalisation, at the request of the patient; and the abolition of the obligation to put into the criminal record the measures with which a judge ordered the hospitalisation of a person in a psychiatric hospital and the revocation of the same.

Although with some limitations, the Mariotti Law represented the landmark between the so-called guardianship phase, in which forced hospitalisation was largely used and the therapeutic role was something marginal, and the so-called sanitary phase, a proper therapeutic phase in which forced hospitalisation was not something primary and sometimes became a sort of instrument for cure (Scarcella et al., 1980).

In 1969 the psychiatric hospital of Cogoleto became autonomous and later was divided in different areas, that is, each pavilion or a group of pavilions housed patients from a specific geographic area of the province of Savona and part of the province of Genoa. Among the effects of this division was the cessation of monthly "deportations" of unwanted patients from the hospital in Quarto. Patients waiting for admission were no longer concentrated in the so-called observation pavilion: they were distributed among all departments. They were no longer distinguished according to pathological features but area of origin.

The "sectoralisation" of the psychiatric hospital was inspired by the French model of hospitalisation. It aimed to guarantee therapeutic continuity between the services in a patient's hometown and the hospital. Unfortunately, this brought another element of degradation to Italian psychiatric hospitals: the mixture of different pathologies and difficulty in planning therapeutic and rehabilitative programs for individuals and groups.

The indisputable opposition to the subdivision of institutional space into wards for agitated, calm, and ill-gotten people led to a diagnostic carelessness due to its excessive sociological reductionism. A consequence was a therapeutic-rehabilitative and prognostic carelessness that provoked a downward indistinction, a distorted egalitarianism for all patients without any perspective and hope.

The Mariotti Law established some forms of voluntary release from a psychiatric facility. In this phase, physicians and nurses showed more interest towards patients and their conditions, so an aid and ambulatorial network was created. Although underdeveloped, it was more efficient than what existed before.

In 1929, the first neuropsychiatric regional clinic of Genoa was opened at Sampierdarena, a popular and proletarian area and thus particularly appropriate for this experiment.

The organisational transformations that can be put under the expression "sector psychiatry" did not radically modify the punitive and guardianship ideology. This ideology is still at the basis of the existence itself of the psychiatric hospital (De Salvia, 1977).

The daily conditions of the hospitalised did not change. Many of them remained physically restrained night and day. The aberrant practice of lobotomy for the agitated did not stop (although it was limited to exceptional cases) as well as the undiscriminated and sadistic use of electroshock. Internal spaces remained narrow, hygienic conditions more distressing than precarious, and connection with the outside scarce and limited to those few cases classified as non-chronic.

The 1960s represented the zenith of asylum culture but also the beginning of its decline.

In 1978, the activities and theories of Franco Basaglia (1981–1982) and his coworkers, which radically criticised the existence itself of the asylums, permitted to promulgate Law 180 (known as the Basaglia Law), later included in Law 833 of the Sanitary Reformation. This declared the end of the asylums. It was a framework law with a strong provocative power and an important utopian vision that had a significant influence of praxes, habits, and prejudices. Its difficult realisation touched important points of civil cohabitation, more precisely those about the criteria of danger, mental disease, personal freedom, and exploitation (De Martis, 1987).

Following the guiding principle of the right of the patient to "response to need" rather than the purported danger they posed to society, Law 180 established that all psychiatric hospitals in the country could no longer accept new admissions.

This was the genesis of psychiatric services of diagnosis and cure in public hospitals and mental health services. There were more attempts to prevent mental distress and to offer relief from the most acute moments of suffering, but the longer-lasting aspects of mental disease were hastily and generically classified as chronic and clearly less considered.

The Basaglia Law caused bewilderment and even panic in many psychiatrists and public opinion. This was probably due to the widespread feeling of being unarmed in front of the new challenge of madness: the loss of the asylum, the physical place that could treat it "on behalf of the normal people," became concrete (Giacanelli, 1975).

The law called for the construction of structures alternative to hospitalisation. Unfortunately, the features of these structures were not defined as well as the time and cost it would take to create them.

After an enthusiastic and often ideological increase in the number of resignations from psychiatric hospitals, the incompleteness of the legislative framework forced workers to slow down. In fact, Italy did not have either those structures or the means necessary to receive and contain people.

The conditions of psychiatry appeared chaotic throughout Italy. In particular, the psychiatric services of public hospitals in Liguria were filled with hospitalisations defined as improper. This was not an expression of the acuteness of the clinical features of different diseases; rather, it was the expression of a social emergency and an absence of alternatives to hospitalisation in a psychiatric ward.

Mental health services aimed to respond to the demands of psychiatric hospitalisation but, without efficacious tools, they excessively pushed for patients to return to their families. Because of the lack of personnel and the great difficulty of the task, mental services could not guarantee continuous or adequate support to the patients' families. In the absence of the state proposing a good and innovative law, all the burden fell on families.

Because of the weakness of the new services and lack of adequate funding, in May 1983 the Liguria government (that, in the meantime, acquired authority on psychiatry) made it possible for a patient to return to the former psychiatric hospital, that would be called Presidio Sociale e Sanitario per la Tutela della Salute Mentale (social and health care centre for the protection of mental health). This applied to those patients who were hospitalised at least once in a psychiatric hospital or a judicial psychiatric hospital before December 1981.

The 1983 law was written and established to counter the great risks of abandonment of patient who resigned from the former psychiatric institute.

A 1988 regional law abolished every temporal limit concerning the return to the hospital, considering the impossibility of a hospitalisation in the social and health care district for those patients who never lived in a psychiatric hospital.

The legislative transformation of the psychiatric hospital into a social and health care district, which promised a therapeutic-rehabilitative service for those patients wanting to enter again, coincided with the institutional disinterest towards the therapeutic function. There was a formal and legislative reality dealing with the rehabilitation and the therapeutic continuity and a substantial reality making the social and health care district the heir of the psychiatric hospital. Of course, although this district did not have the most violent and barbaric features of the asylums, it featured high levels of illegality and indignity.

The high number of readmissions of relatively young patients stressed the great limits of the hypothesis of a quick closure of psychiatric hospitals.

The idea of a former asylum transformed into a place for old and long-term patients was largely refuted by the data of three studies (Schinaia et al., 1991, 1993, 1996), which showed that the social and health care district became a "terminal institutional dump" for people from other "dumps" such retirement homes and psychiatric hospitals for criminals.

The high number of readmissions should have given meaning to the therapeutic function. This function could have taken place inside a properly planned social and health care district, one based on community rules, waiting for new projects to overcome the concept of asylum. This was supposed to transfer the assistance functions to more suitable structures in the communities to which the patients belonged. Unfortunately, the administrations and the politics appeared to completely forget these points.

The hygienic conditions got even worse, the walls and the environmental structures more obsolete, the personnel (especially the nursing staff) more reduced. Psychologists and social workers were not hired; the lack of financial investments and political projects had as a consequence the abandonment of working hypothesis of therapy and rehabilitation, independently from the continuous anti-entropic efforts of the staff.

The type of asylum that had to disappear by law remained, but it was as if it were not there. Once again, we witnessed the great repression of the asylum, "the land of abandonment." As long as a minimal residual of the asylum will remain, even if encysted and closed to the novelty, it will remain an open wound, which will not closed spontaneously (De Martis et al., 1980).

The intervention of the anti-adulteration unit of the Carabinieri was necessary to letting the public know that the district resembled the stronghold in *The Tartar Steppe* (1940) of Dino Buzzati. There was very few to hold in a place that became the desert of communication and emotions. The unit discovered serious irregularities, from the abuse of restraint means to the abandonment of disabled people, in an environment and structures that were severely degraded due to an absence of regular maintenance over two decades. After an inspection, the examining magistrate declared some wards to be "human warehouses."

In 1993, the administration and the head of the social and health care district changed so that the most degraded ward was closed. The first secure residential community was launched. The readmissions were stopped and new projects to restore the wards and the social centre were presented. The living conditions of the patients and the general environmental conditions improved. The hope started to return to that far hill of Pratozanino, where the Cogoleto Psychiatric Hospital was built, and in which a long time ago it was decided to hide mental suffering from the public eye.

It appeared to be possible to give value in these "dead souls" a so rich heritage of humanity: a heritage full of meanings, disturbing questions, and radical messages for the crucial areas of the human experience: all things that represent a source of spiritual enrichment and precious reflection (De Martis et al., 1980).

2 Thinking Beyond the Asylum

Although the Basaglia Law, or Law 180, of 1978 prescribed the definitive closure of asylums, most of these institutions remained for a long time, along with all their environmental degradation, anti-therapeutic segregation, and inhuman abandon.

Thus, a new law in 1994 reconfirmed the closure of the former asylums and set a new deadline of December 31, 1996.

This new mandate supported all the initiatives previously started by the asylums amidst many difficulties. It also forced the public administrations that failed to follow them to finally plan accordingly, despite the risk that doing so would reduce the national health-care budget, a risk that became reality. There was another painful reality: many of the idealistic dimensions of the plan were never put in place.

The guidelines for replacing the asylums, defined by the monitoring unit of the Italian Ministry of Health in 1996, specified that this be accomplished by some means other than throwing the patients out. It was considered necessary to avoid transformations unable to truly change the institutional situation, and mass transmigrations to public or private facilities for chronic conditions such as long-term care, pensioners, assisted living residences, and orthophrenic institutes. These facilities were deemed unable to guarantee the right to real help and needed rehabilitative interventions. It was mandatory to think about personalised rehabilitative projects for those people still living in the former asylums—to consider the duration of their hospitalisations, their personal histories, the history of their diseases, the degree of their present disability, their real possibility of recovery, and their personal and familial resources. Deinstitutionalisation and rehabilitation had to occur through strong collaboration and shared responsibility between the operational unit working in the former asylums and that of the regional services of the national health-care department. An important step was the definition of special operational protocols.

Motivated by the 1996 deadline, some psychiatrists, administrators, and architects devised an ambitious project for transforming the asylum of Cogoleto, which had been both the largest and the most degraded (in

DOI: 10.4324/9781003381723-2

terms of assistance, logistics, and type of patients) asylum in central and northern Italy.

Any such project is between Scylla and Charybdis, that is, it must consider two opposite risks: first, an ideological trust in the capacity of the institution to self-consume because it is experienced as non-transformable and thus irreducible to any project except its natural extinction; second, the faith in the structural and technological modernisation of the asylum because it would dress up the new system in the same excluding and segregating dynamics of the old asylum.

Furthermore, a viable project must consider the financial budget, not only for the present but also for the future. The project must be sustainable and able to guarantee a function of assistance over time: it must go beyond the former residents of the old asylum and support new patients who had never experienced the bad old days.

The plan for Cogoleto set as its goal to avoid every risk related to the idea of a new asylum. It aimed to be polyfunctional and multidisciplinary.

An intense anti-institutional effort allowed a good part of patients to be discharged quite quickly: they did not require 24-hour health assistance but only psychosocial rehabilitation interventions in regional structures. Very few were able to return to live with their families. Most went to family-like setting (groups of no more of ten in apartments or communities hosting no more than 20).

For patients who could not be discharged in the short term it was necessary to organise a rehabilitative intervention to overcome the difficulties caused by the long hospitalisation and be reintegrated in society.

In the final years, nurses, social workers, and psychiatrists of the former asylum of Cogoleto transformed the old model of the closed psychiatric ward into a community-focused organisation. They opened the doors, making it possible to walk across the spaces. They guaranteed progressively higher levels of privacy, improved clothing and food, and created groups for playing, working, and thinking. Patients could make more trips to visit museums, the cinema, and the theatre. They could hone and express their specific individual skills through painting, ceramics, sculpture, gardening lessons, singing in choirs, dance, gymnastics, and sports such as soccer and horse riding. Parties attracted many visitors with the relative possibility of sharing experiences and meeting with the families of the guests (the new name for the patients) to manage daily life and discuss future plans.

All this drastically reduced the population. Only nine of the 19 wards built at the beginning of the 20th century were still functioning. Several therapeutic-rehabilitative communities were established in the city from 1997 to 1999, each with no more than 20 people, all adequately assisted around the clock.

The main aim of these efforts was to guarantee to the patients the possibility to return to Genoa, where they could find themselves again, meet and talk with other people, and be citizens among other citizens. Genoa is not and cannot be the idealised end after a long stay in the institution. It is not only the city of the sea and beautiful houses, artistic and tourist attractions, and civil coexistence: it is also the city of drug addiction, closing down factories, youth unemployment, chaotic traffic, and pollution.

It is a vital crossing of open contradictions, contrasting with the deadly flattening of the atmosphere of the asylum.

The asylum had always been depicted as the last landfill and final collector not only of crazy people but also of demented elderly ripped away from their families and psychophysical disabled of varied severity. The disabled comprised one-third of the patient population of Cogoleto, and the geriatric residents the other third.

After a long period in which psychiatrists treated these groups inadequately—that is, based on repression and guardianship—there should have followed an intensive period of restructuring, of forming multi-professional operational units composed of psychiatrists, psychologists, neurologists, and physiatrists who could affect soma-psyche integration and human curing. The distinction of patients in three categories (elderly, disabled, and actual psychiatric patients) represented an important step towards civilisation because it destroyed the amalgam of institutional confusion that, similarly to the Hegelian night of the world, made all the cows black and allowed a more significant personalisation of the rehabilitative projects.

Another effort was to put on the market both the considerable but unused real estate assets and those assets that would progressively no longer be used, to finance the reconversion projects. Buildings and areas that were not expected to be used again would be sold only at the condition that they would be directed to other functions compatible with those assistance and sanitary activities conducted in the former asylum. The profits would finance the construction of structures that would replace the asylums.

The housing project would have been utterly incomplete if it did not include recreational and rehabilitative spaces such as a community centre (perhaps the central place of the projects thanks to its unifying all the paths), some art rooms for painting, pottery, and crafts (with the collaboration of local artistic high schools), sports grounds (with a football field that non-residents could use), and an auditorium and theatre for choir, dance, and dramatic expression (Schinaia, 1998a).

To avoid isolation, a therapeutic and rehabilitative area was envisioned in the immense available green space, in which the health-care authority and social cooperatives could work together.

The agricultural lands of the asylum were quite extensive and represented a natural and landscape heritage in the Ligurian Riviera. The quality of the soil (because it was left fallow for decades), the midday sun exposure, and the mild climate of the Ligurian Sea favour the cultivation of typical Mediterranean vegetation: maritime pines, olive and fruit trees, vegetables, and spices. The transformation of this land into a productive agricultural area could have guaranteed work for at least 15 people and helped to re-socialise people back to all parts of the region.

The therapeutic and rehabilitative project wanted to address:

a the problem of youth employment in a particularly acute phase of social crisis
b the challenge of reintegrating and psychiatric patients
c the possibility of socialising elderly people
d the need to safeguard the natural heritage of the area, through the reuse of the "ecological oasis," which madness saved from consumerism and allotment.

The work activities would include farmyard animal breeding, organic food production, animal husbandry, running horse stables, beekeeping, and marketing products, but also agritourism such as catering and hospitality activities, a botanical garden, and nature trails.

The more the experience of going beyond the asylum was connected to the external—to a real, concrete contradictory but not idealised and ideological external—the more the projects could be realised and provide individual therapeutic work, a relationship with the suffering subject, a containment of psychotic anxieties, and all the things that are preparatory to each program of psychosocial rehabilitation.

3 Projects and Materials for a Nativity Scene in the Asylum

In the early 1980s, the hopes fuelled by Basaglia Law, or Law 180, of 1978 gave way to disillusionment and discouragement throughout Italy. The lack of interest for patients and their care was increasingly evident at the political and administrative level. The health-care workers felt as abandoned as their patients, like keepers of a place without any affective or economic investment. Inert and detached spectators of the inhuman agony of the asylum, overwhelmed by the ongoing degradation and lack of enthusiasm, settled for giving mere routine help.

It was at this low moment that a group of health-care workers and patients felt the need to plan a nativity scene representing the individual and institutional suffering and the way it took shape throughout the years—a plastic expression of memory, a sort of *genius loci* attesting to the features and peculiarities of the asylum and impeding the gestures and actions to distort its real nature and history.

The artistic creativity in asylums and psychiatric hospitals started to be scientifically recognised by the psychiatrist and art historian Hans Prinzhorn in his 1922 book *Bildnerei der Geisteskranken. Ein Beitrag zur Psychologie und Psychopathologie der Gestaltung* (*Artistry of the Mentally Ill: A Contribution to the Psychology and Psychopathology of Configuration*). In his introduction to the French edition (1984), Jean Starobinski argues that the works produced in asylums can be interpreted as artistic *tout court*, rather than only as a kind of exotic art comparable to the primitive arts and to be placed behind the display cases protecting relics of the past.

The story of the Nativity Scene at the Cogoleto asylum started in 1980: it was decided to transfer the experience and atmosphere of the crèche that was created every year in each pavilion to a central location under the supervision of nurses and nuns. The aim was to build a unique and permanent scene for the entire hospital. The chosen spot was the basement of the pavilion in which the typography studio had once been, a central area easily accessible to everyone.

After many lively discussions it was decided that the scene should be set in the everyday life of the 1960s: it was rightly considered the time of the paradigmatic expression of the life inside the asylum in its crude and

DOI: 10.4324/9781003381723-3

brutal (and protected by the silence of the surrounding countryside and woods) reality.

The most important local nativity scenes were visited to find the best operational solution for creating one in Cogoleto. At last, a structure composed of a series of representations was chosen, a long sequence of sketches on each of the two sides of a winding corridor.

By having to walk through a corridor in order to view the Nativity Scene, the spectator experienced the physical and mental sensations of a progressive penetration into a largely unknown world, characterised by its own laws. Navigating a labyrinth of mind and dexterity was a formidable way to instill in the spectator that tangle of emotions and feelings (not only anxiety and pain but also hope, curiosity, and solidarity) at the base of the relationships inside the institutional microcosm.

Patients, nurses, and physicians exchanged information and traded technical and professional notions. Tomaso Molinari, a capable and enthusiastic nurse trying to put together the different contributions without distorting or misunderstanding but even exalting them, supervised the entire creation process. Bruno Galati created most of the statuettes and the settings: a young worker in the psychiatric hospital, he later became a hyperrealist artist specialising in terracotta works.

The involvement of the patients in every part of the creation, from the choice of location to the planning of the representations, was the central pillar of the project. With the help of hospital staff, the patients searched for the materials, such as branches, boughs, no longer used fabrics, polystyrene, and generic waste, all found within the asylum walls.

The spaces were cleared out; tables, counters, and everything that could serve as a surface were placed along the walls; the infrastructure was erected with poles and tree trunks taken from the surrounding woods; the vault of the gallery was made with branches and bamboo canes. Polystyrene sheets were used to delimit the sectors; many newspapers were glued together to create hillsides; many large sheets of paper smeared with various colours and glued together were used for the external cladding of the infrastructure. Branches were cut from the hedges and olive trees to recreate the gardens; the internal scenography was composed of wood furniture in polystyrene and statuettes partly in earthenware and partly in papier-mâché with their core made of wire and covered with various fabrics from the nurses' gowns and the nuns' habits. A complex electrical system made for a suggestive play of lights.

People who worked at the hospital were proud to voluntarily participate in some manner to the setting up of the Nativity Scene and, above all, to represent their real-life activity in the institution.

Thus, the Nativity Scene was made of representations such as the treasure's cash office or the syndicate's room. These places could be dismissed as insignificant at a first glance, but they were not. In fact, the patients felt them to as the central places of power, so highly meaningful and deserving of representation.

Some patients spontaneously organised taking turns to keep watch over the crèche, which evoked ancient affective images and rooted family traditions in them, from the aggression of other, less autonomous, and controlled patients.

During the creation of the Nativity Scene, between planning and construction, many patients withdrew from the project, so tremendous was their anxiety and discomfort when they realised that the work represented the place of their sufferings. They ran away horrified and scared: for the first time, they could see their intolerable life and unacceptable misery from an external point of view. The idea that the crèche was a place of death and not of memory was circulated among them. Later, many of them refused to enter it, limiting themselves to turning around it with curiosity.

The Nativity Scene of Cogoleto asylum was inaugurated in 1984 after *circa* four years of intense and continuous work. It must be understood as a representation, a tangible expression, and translation of a religious feeling rooted in a spontaneous motion toward faith, not as the reductive formula of minor artistic expression. It is a sort of static theatre leaving more space to the natural than to idealisation and devotion.

In the *Enciclopedia dello Spettacolo* (Encyclopaedia of Performing Arts) (1961), Stefanucci defines the crèche as a tridimensional representation of the birth of Jesus created with mobile figures and veristic elements (such as houses, rocks, plants, etc.) for Christmas and without reference to Purification. It is connected with the history of theatre because it aims to render real and present an event far in space and time through a spectacular fiction. This definition stresses the feature of scenic fiction, showing that creating a crèche requires the use of scenographic elements (such as backdrops or natural elements), sound and light, and, of course, statuettes-characters. In this sense, the crèche can be interpreted as a miniature stage (Sommariva, 1993).

The choice to represent the institutional sufferance by creating a big crèche, the result of collective work, was determined by the evocative force of the Nativity. This is the privileged place of childhood and family memories with a simple construction that unites various cultural stories. Through direct contact with the work, spectators can recognise themselves in it and find elements of social and cultural affinity easily at the emotional and psychological level. They can feel dumbfounded and enchanted when enclosed in the scenography of the crèche and even become actors of a "living" human landscape (Bettanini and Moreno, 1970).

There are signs that the Nativity was represented in the third through fourth centuries in a frescoed niche with the Madonna, Child, and three Magi in the Catacombs of Domitilla in Rome and in the fourth to sixth centuries in the reliefs of the sarcophagi in which Saint Joseph and the

Shepherd appear. The crèche as a plastic and tridimensional representation is rooted in the spectacular matrix of the Sacred Representations and the *Laudes* that, since the early Middle Ages, were set up in churchyards and confraternities with the typical arrangement of scenes. Certain actions deferred over time were interpreted simultaneously.

Thomas of Celano points out that in 1223, Saint Francis of Assisi prepared the Christmas vigil in the grotto of Greccio. Villagers came and lit up the night with lights and candles. The crèche (in ancient Latin *praesepium*) was filled with straw and a real ox and a real donkey were placed on its sides. Mary and Joseph were not represented. The novel aspect was that the crèche was put outside churches and became part of an actual landscape in an authentic winter night. Gone was the separation between the stage and stalls: here was a sacred drama in which farmers and shepherds with their flocks interpreted themselves and acted as background actors.

The idea that Saint Francis of Assisi invented the crèche is no longer reliable today. Nonetheless, it is indisputable that the Franciscan crèche had a crucial historical value: it was a paradigmatic example of spontaneous and popular religiousness and a break in the inflexibility of the rituality of the Church. In fact, for the masses living the faith in a commonsensical manner the presence of a visible image rendered completely useless the intellectual demonstration of the truth of something. In other words, if faith was able to show itself to the people, it was not mandatory for it to be persuasive. Only later, the Baroque crèche, displaying a seducing beauty, introduced the idea of art as a form of persuasion.

The decay of the Sacred Representations, which the Church often considered too secular and profane, allows for the Nativity themes represented in them be expressed in new forms and manners. At the time of the Counter-Reformation, the sacred drama intended as a mimesis occurring in the city streets transformed into something icastic and motionless composed of statues (Riolfo Marengo, 1996).

In 1283 the Gothic era Tuscan sculptor Arnolfo di Cambio created the first crèche with fully sculped characters. It seems that these characters were powerful figures, but today only a few mutilated ones remain in the Church of Santa Maria Maggiore in Rome.

Following a chronological order, the second crèche is that in the Church of Santo Stefano in Bologna. It consists of five full-size wooden figures dating back to 1370 (Buoniconti Aschettino, 1992).

In the 15th and 16th centuries crèches of different shapes can be found, especially in Lombardy and Naples. The 15th century is famous for terracotta. In the crypt of the Cathedral of Modena there are the crèche of Antonio Begarelli and that of the Madonna della Pappa (the Madonna of Food) of Guido Mazzoni, in which a character feeds the Child with a bowl.

Beginning in the 1600s the crèche gradually started to lose its medieval symbolism and started to assume a tridimensional and realistic representation of Nativity by introducing secondary characters.

The golden age of the crèche was the 18th century, when it became a worldwide phenomenon starting in Naples.

The more the 15th century entered the Baroque, the more the crèche assumed an encyclopedic character: all the jobs, all the animals, all the food, all the fruit, and all the vegetables were represented. The crèche became the market: the great symbol of the totality of the world. The characters did not limit themselves to adore the Child: they exhibited themselves or their job and function. This is because here the sacred shows itself to the world and the world to the sacred (Citati, 1997).

In the first 20 years of the 17th century, the statues decreased in proportion, reducing from the natural size to the "triplet," corresponding to about 40 centimeters. However, they increased considerably in number. There was the passage from static to mobile representation by using flexible and articulated mannequins (Borrelli, 1991).

The characters were made of iron mannequins stuffed with fibre. The fact that these baroque statuettes were joined permitted to remove the characters from the crèche every year and to alter their poses according to what the directors of the crèche required for their installation.

These small figures, showing phantasmagorical roles going beyond the meaning of the liturgical event, were placed in fantastic and historically unreliable set-ups.

The head of the statuettes was made of polychromous terracotta, the eyes of crystal, the extremities of wood. The costumes were made of fabric with minuscule drawings.

Every statuette was dressed according to the represented character following the codified features of tradition and according to constant but differentiated types to stress the different role of each. The dresses had a precise symbolic value that could be decodified by considering the overall view of the crèche. The first need was to make immediately perceivable the fact that a certain figure pertained to the realm of divinity or that of humanity.

The crèche appeared as a microcosm in which the miniaturised costumes depicted the fundamental themes of society of that time. The three powers (political, religious, military) having the function of organising social life stressed their superiority by dressing in "uniformised" styles with repeated symbolic elements that everyone could recognise as emblems of power. By contrast, the shepherds, beggars, and female figures realistically represented the variety of dresses of the poor classes (Cataldi Gallo, 1993).

The settings of the crèches tended to realistically reproduce the life of the community of those who planned them. Naturalism was a fundamental feature of 17th-century art considering the crèche as a figurative

genre. In fact, archaeology, ethnography, folklore, theatre (both sophisticated and popular), street, and religious shows, many various emotions
and inspirations converged in the small proscenium of the crèche (Causa,
1987). It was the triumph of most meticulous verism because every tool or
environment represented was built with absolute precision and fidelity.

The Neapolitan crèche was the first typical popular with a background
and landscape. It consists of two parts: the main one, the Mystery, with the
sacred figures of the Madonna, Saint Joseph, and the Child, the Angel,
the ox, and the donkey; and the complementary one, the *Diversorio*, with
the taverns, the annunciation, market, all the places of mundanity,
something disenchanted and secular.

The flight of the Angels must be followed to find the most important
scene, the Nativity. In the spot in which most of the Angels are gathered,
forming a sort of cluster, there is the grotto of the Sacred Family.
Sometimes it is in a marginal position in the lively overall scene.

The crèche is one of the most famous iconographic images that, losing
its original and religious meaning, started to develop a spontaneous
representation related to the world of dreams, folklore, and fairy tales. It
resets the distinction between sky and earth, the sacred and the profane.

In the representation of the Nativity, profane elements found place
and shape into the crèche. These elements were linked to ancient costumes, rites, and myths of peasant culture. It is not by chance that many
characters of the crèches were allegories of other mythological figures of
the pre-Christian culture and spirituality. Two examples are the "black
shepherd," the ancient bringer of misfortune, and the "white shepherd,"
the ancient bringer of grace (Bordignon Elestici, 1991).

The ox and the donkey were two original symbols of Patristic literature,
identifying the former in the Jew and the latter in the Christian, both
adoring the newborn Christ. It is important to note that this is not strongly
confirmed because an evangelic documentation on the crèche is missing.
Only Luke talks of the "manger" and from here it follows that the ico-
nology of the crèche is directly connected to the ancient literary tradition
of the Patristic and Apocryphal Gospels. It is a clear example of how
popular culture assumes the legend of the ox and the donkey and even
maintains the iconological features of the Biblical characters having a
relevant part in the Sacred Representations.

The construction of animated scenes with puppets (*crèches et santons*)
started in Provence relatively late (around the 17th century) and spread
throughout France only a century later (Ripert, 1956). The puppets were
plaster figurines constructed in series and characterised by many vivid
colours. Perhaps they originally came from Italy.

The crèches combined the narratives of the Canonical and Apocryphal
Gospels and the narrative of everyday facts and gossips. There were extremely widespread, but the profane features came over the sacred ones:
the scenes passed from the sacrifice of Isaac to a representation of a thief

robbing a man getting his shoes shined. The religious authorities opposed this custom, but nonetheless it survived for centuries. The puppeteers were expelled from the churches yet they continued to hold their shows in miserable small theatres or the streets. This custom lasted until permission to perform sacred representations with puppets was denied to everyone in every place. From that moment, marionettes and puppets were abandoned and often donated to churches: they were deprived of strings and voice and used to replace the life-size statues of the large nativity scenes of the previous centuries.

If the tradition of the popular crèche was mainly developed in the furnaces of unknown Ligurian potters and freely inspired the design of the single figurines, then the Nativity Scene of Cogoleto has its cultural roots in the Neapolitan crèche and Provençal marionettes. The main difference between them is the way in which the social sphere is represented. In the Neapolitan crèche and in the *crèches provençales*, every reference to this sphere is simply anecdotal, representing an everyday life distant from the dramatic event of Nativity. The characters are often benevolent, kind, and happy. The picturesque serenity of the scenography gives the idea that everything can be repaired and work at the social level, so that it transmits a sort of manic and denialist feeling. On the contrary, the Nativity Scene of Cogoleto immediately presents the social sphere in light of its irrefutable tragedy. This coincides with the symbolic event of the birth of Christ. It does not aim to comfort or make room for narcissistic fascination. It shows the pain from unusual perspectives and makes it immediately perceivable. It reveals the condition of patients without defensive masks and provokes contradictory feelings in the spectator: closeness and estrangement, admiration and annoyance, curiosity and restlessness. As an artistic expression, it allows the project to combine the religious (through the theme of Nativity) and the social (through the painful and extremely realistic representation of the outcasts). The result is a commemoration, sometimes merciless, sometimes vaguely nostalgic, of everyday life in the asylum, like a concentration camp, with its many contradictory aspects. Thus, it is a sort of document, a memory, and a testimony, giving a global vision of institutional life, reproducing the forced routine of the various moments in the patients' lives. It shows their ordeal as well as the roles of the physicians and nurses, both accomplices and victims of the institutional deterioration.

The Nativity Scene of Cogoleto offers a good amalgam of cathartic and pedagogical functions, of the defensive and self-observational.

To reach the Nativity Scene a gate must be crossed and then, after passing through an opening that seems to be carved into stone, a corridor on the walls of which polystyrene panels are hung. On these panels are the large factory, port, cultivated countryside, city of Genoa, a town of the Ligurian hinterland—the "life" and the "outside" of the 16,000 patients who lived in those places and then lived in that asylum. Two larger panels follow, representing Genoa with its lighthouse and Savona with its *torretta*

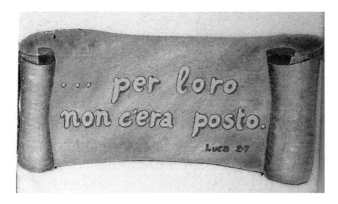

Figure 3.1 The lettering at the entrance of the Nativity Scene.

(little tower), that is, the cities from which most of the patients came. The beautiful wording placed at the entrance of the crèche itself warns, "There was no room for them" (Figure 3.1). It is a clear reference to Luke's gospel verse (II-7) that reads, "She wrapped him in cloths and placed him in a manger, because there was no guest room available for them." A patient suggested this reference when she said that "The Virgin Mary was not accepted in a hotel because she was pregnant and a pregnant woman is always a source of problems. All the people avoid her. This is what happened to me: I was a source of many problems for my family that had no other chance than closing me in here." Only a great task can justify the renouncement of personal freedom, hopes, and existence: on the contrary, enduring internment in an asylum could be intolerable. Mary was refused and driven out, but gave birth to the son of God and thus received a reward for her enormous sufferings.

The identification with the Virgin Mary allowed this patient to justify her suffering through the repression of her basic needs and the sublimation of her drives, faithfully waiting for a fantastic event or a compensatory future gratification.

The Nativity Scene has the function of a ritual that always repeats itself in the same way. It can reassure because its conclusion can be predicted. But this reassurance must not be intended as a form of anaesthesia—that is, a passive adjustment to the rules of the asylum—but as a form of basic survival of the Self, a persisting and perturbing resistance to institutional decay. It is a patient and reparative opposition to the renouncing and the feeling of impotence.

The Nativity Scene gives everyone the chance to stop, look back to the past, and think, not to find a reflection in the deforming mirror of a past only apparently quiet and orderly, but to continue the interrupted path with more motivation, more collaboration, and more certain of our goals.

4   The Nativity

For the Catholic religion, a child, the son of God, born from a virgin mother and set down in a manger, came with the mission to save mankind from evil through his sacrifice and death.

The history of religions is full of natal events, prodigious births of divine men whose destiny is to save the world.

Emanations of light and appearances of stars announced the birth of the Buddha; the fulgor of a new comet revealed Bethlehem's grotto to the Magi; in Greek mythology, many births, such as those of Zeus and Heracles, were hailed as miracles.

The myth of the birth of the hero (Rank, 1909) presents a common narrative: the hero is the son of important parents, often of a king or divinity. Many difficulties precede his conception, for example, extended infertility or the duty to keep secret the sexual union between the father and mother. Before or during the pregnancy, a prophecy, dream, or oracle warns about the risks surrounding his birth, more precisely, that it would endanger the life of the father. Thus, the newborn is often put in a container which is then set on the water and he is saved by people of an inferior social rank or female animals. When he reaches adulthood, he finds his real parents. The prophecy is fulfilled. He is recognised and can receive the honours due to him.

Otto Rank interprets this mythical narrative, which includes the birth of Christ, as phantasies, which Freud classified under the term "family romance." The child imagines that the couple who live with him are not his real parents, that he was born of much more important parents and that his so-called parents merely adopted or hosted him; or, as an alternative, that the alleged father is not his actual parent and that, by definition, his mother had a clandestine relationship (Freud, 1909).

As we can see, a psychoanalytic interpretation confirms that the centre of the crèche is the iconographic place and representation of childish phantasies.

On the right of the Nativity Scene of the Cogoleto asylum is the first big scene representing the Nativity (Figure 4.1). Unlike the other scenes of the

DOI: 10.4324/9781003381723-4

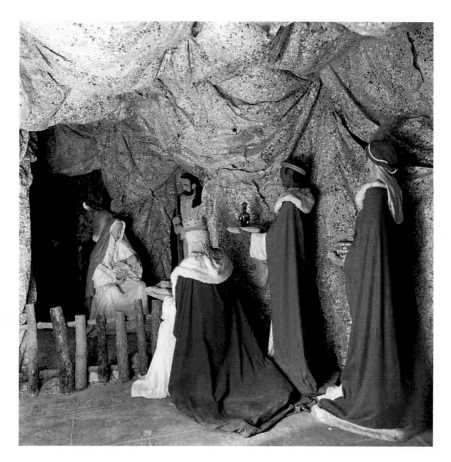

Figure 4.1 The Nativity.

crèche, all the figures are full size in order to immediately express the relevance of the themes of birth, family belonging, and the mother-child relationship.

Papier-mâché figures of Mary and Joseph show faces with marked traits, dark eyes, and hair, which reveal the South Italian origin of its creator and many inpatients.

There is a clear scenographic difference when compared to the oleographic representation of traditional and popular crèches: the Child, who has a snotty face, is not put down in a manger; he stays in his mother's arms, wrapped in a veil on her chest, and gazes into her eyes (Figure 4.2).

The Madonna does not carry the typical virginal expression of the traditional iconography: she has the hard and absorbed look of a peasant woman who has just breastfed and holds the newborn in her arms, waiting for it to fall asleep (Figure 4.3).

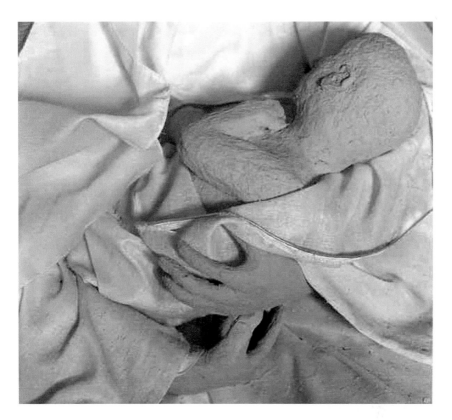

Figure 4.2 The Nativity (detail).

It is common to see the Child completely wrapped in a veil, with his face hidden from view. It is a scenographic choice, which had not been planned: it stresses the need not only for confidentiality but also for exclusivity, something that the experience of the asylum brutally denies.

The expression "only the mother can see the child in the eyes," coined by an inpatient and often repeated by many others as a sort of mantra, highlights the need for a place in which individual memories and phantasies can settle. It is the opposite of the collective flattening of memories that impend the chance of self-recognition.

The grotto is a symbol of the limit between the inside and the outside: inside it, the Child is still grabbed onto the maternal body to which he was omnipotently united and must face for the first time the pain of completely depending on the Other, on the external world. He is between the incommensurable nostalgia of the past and suffering reality of the present.

The issue of the trauma of birth probably caused the rupture of the relationship between Rank and Freud. Rank (1924) argued that birth is the

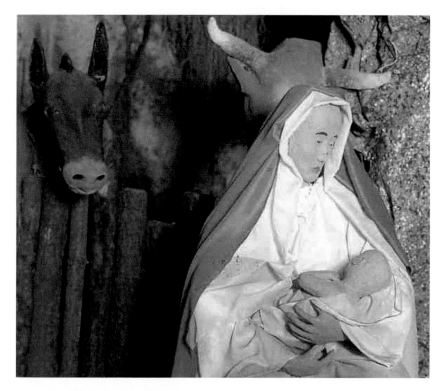

Figure 4.3 The Nativity (detail).

first experience and prototype of anxiety, specifically separation anxiety, whereas Freud (1926) posited that the trauma of birth is something biological, not psychological because we cannot know everything about the mental states of the foetus or how it experiences suffering. For him, *at birth no object existed and so no object could be missed* (Freud, 1926, p. 170).

Melanie Klein, Donald Winnicott, Eugenio Gaddini, and all the later studies in the field of infant observation show that the difference between Rank and Freud's views is not so significative. They recognise the reality of the physical character of the first emotional experiences of the newborn, but they distinguish these experiences from anxiety as adults feel it, thus avoiding shifts towards adultomorphic theories in which the child is thought of as an adult.

Winnicott (1949) proposes three categories of experience about birth. In the first category, postulated *a priori* and not demonstrated, there is a kind of normal and healthy experience, a valid and positive but limited experience because it is so infrequent. It establishes a natural model of living and can be reinforced by other subsequent normal experiences. The experience of birth is an important factor of a favourable sequence leading to the development of trust, sense of continuity, stability, safety, etc.

In the second category there is the common experience of the moderately traumatic birth that is later connected to different traumatic environmental factors. It reinforces them and, in turn, is reinforced by them.

In the third category, there is the extreme case of traumatic experience that subsequent cures cannot repair in any manner.

Birth is the first great separation. The total and exclusive contact, the symbiosis between mother and child break off painfully. Depressive suffering is a peculiar quality of the human species that starts from birth, when for the first time the newborn feels less pressure, a sort of depression and thus a depression, due to the loss of the bodily containment of the maternal womb (Carloni, 1984).

The pain is in the birth pangs and in the cries of the child, who abandons the warm and protective maternal womb to venture towards the external open world.

The mind starts functioning at birth when the newborn is exposed at the most important physiological upheaval of his existence. Suddenly, everything changes for the foetus: breathing becomes pulmonary; the surrounding environment is no longer liquid and uniform in temperature; the impact with air and loss of continuous contact mean the loss of a constant and safe limit (the uterine wall) that, until then, had been the natural border of the foetus.

The child is physically but not mentally separated from the mother. After the birth, he will continue to be unable to feel the difference between himself and the outside world. A part of what the child believes is his body is actually the maternal body (as it was originally the uterine wall), but for him it is part of his body, a border of himself. In the child's mind, there is no mother distant from him but an always available mother who immediately satisfies his every need.

The child cannot understand that the breast does not belong him. He simply experiences sensations that stop the tension, but imagines himself able to produce everything by himself only. The surrounding world is merely a product of his magical omnipotence.

Psychological birth occurs five or six months after biological birth. The child begins to comprehend his status of absolute dependence on an outside world, that he cannot understand and manage in any way. The mind grasps the destruction of the magical and omnipotent world upon which the feeling of Self was based.

The outside acquires a terrible power and the child has the mental sense of a serious mutilation of the Self and the feeling of having failed to survive (Gaddini, 1985; LImentani and Gaddini, 1992).

The first rites of passage serve to integrate the child in the society and reintegrate the mother, who had been temporarily and partially excluded from society after the pregnancy and birth. These rites imply three subsequent stages: separation, border, and aggregation. The child, as well as the stranger, must be separated from the previous world, which is simply his mother.

In general, rites of separation comprise those in which something is cut, for example, a haircut. The rites of aggregation are those having the effect of introducing the child to the world and, among them, the rites of naming, ritual breastfeeding, first dentition, and baptism (Van Gennep, 1909).

The manger is the symbol of nutrition: the adoration of the Magi, who came from afar to offer their gifts symbolising knowledge, recalls the intense anticipation of the birth.

The visit of the Magi to the grotto can be compared to the Platonic cave. The real child to pay homage to is nature and the universe with their deep mysteries (the grotto) and their beauty (Lussana, 1994).

The coming into the world from a grotto is an event that Christianity celebrates every December 25, but it was well known before in the Asian and Greek-Roman world. In fact, in the same day, it was celebrated the birth of Mithra, the Indo-European god of light, who guarantees oaths, is the guardian of truth and adversary of lies. He moves from the darkness of the earth to the brightness of the sky. Light is the symbol of both Mithra and Jesus. But perhaps it is also the symbol of every human being who, at birth, must "come into light" from that "darkness" that is the maternal womb, the cave where we are all conceived for a birth, that birth which alone is not enough and thus calls for a rebirth to find meaning. The feasts of Mithra and of Jesus reaffirm that symbolic vertigo where each one must become his own cave: it is a dark night that has the new day in sight, the so-called *dies natalis* (Galimberti, 1996).

The ox and the donkey give that warmth which, at birth, the Child had to give up and without which he could not survive; Saint Joseph becomes the object of primary paranoia, and in this way he cleanses from violence the mother-child space, showing himself as the paternal guardian of the serenity of the couple (Fornari, 1981). The Child with his mother, the newborn-with-a-breast, is the object of aesthetic apprehension in front of which every man feels love and fear: it is the aesthetic conflict (Meltzer and Harris Williams, 1988).

Images of the Nativity, along with all the other ones representing the scenes of people's everyday life, have the general meaning of the operations of social repairing made for dealing with the drama of birth.

The god becoming a human being through suffering, the omnipotent child becoming cold and helpless and thus dependent but also forcefully dynamic, are metaphors of the human being as a symbolic animal (Cassirer, 1944) who can transform pain and trauma in a cognitive system, in a knowledge process.

The Nativity scene is the place in which all the idealising and sublimating projection of the inpatients occurs. It is the representation of their nostalgia, in those moments in which they can remember, think back to, or imagine their birth.

The strongest motivation behind the desire to go back into the uterus is the search for happiness in the most perfect and unique form we knew (Fodor, 1950).

The inevitable primitive separation from the mother's body makes the child experience the first failure of his narcissistic omnipotence, for which the Ego deforms itself in an idealising manner so it can bear the rejection of the lost beatitude. Nostalgia represents the compensation from the loss of the fusional love (Oneroso Di Lisa, 1989).

Carloni (1989) writes about a prenatal lost paradise characterised by fusional links, in which the garden of Eden is the mother's body that contained all of us, in which children imagine their little unborn brothers in a state of perpetual beatitude. In other words, it is a uterine Nirvana from which everyone of us is expelled. The fall is irreversible and it begins with the cutting of the umbilical cord that connected us to our mother's body.

There is also a neonatal heaven on earth in the mother's arms. It is the only place where we can come back, a pre-oedipal paradise, a place without difficulties, in which we can ignore death and use the language of emotions, a language of poses, gestures, mimicries; a language of attention towards the sensory stimuli more like that of animals than that of adults.

The avid eyes of the child, that get lost in the loving eyes of the mother, give the spectator of the crèche the sensation of a great idealisation but also, in contrast, make palpable the distance between the sweetness of the first scene and the crude realism of the subsequent ones.

5   Segregation

The scenes of the crèche of the asylum coming after that of the Nativity do not deal with reparation or social integration in any way. In fact, they represent neither exclusion nor alienation but the dramatic issue of segregation. Solitude and abandon pervade all the scenes: something surreal and vaguely metaphysical surrounds the statuettes in spaces that the game of lights and perspectives renders gigantic and inadequate for the exchange of words and affections. All of this does not simply set off the idea of separation: it transforms and fixes it in a timeless exclusion.

In the scene representing the gate of the asylum, which is always closed (Figure 5.1), there is the visible manifestation of the neat separation of inside and outside, between what is closed and what is open. The communicative caesura is total and there is no room for dialogue between two irremediably divided worlds.

The mother is far away, absent, lost too soon and traumatically. Her presence is substituted by the theatre of exclusion occurring by maintaining childhood dependence until death, the fear of autonomy and being confused with the other.

With its false scaffolding, the rigid and cold institution only appears to make up for the absence of the father—the "social third" allowing the transformation of the pain of separation into a form of knowledge through his evolutive containment.

By crucial default, perhaps a clear failure, of the separation processes, the primitive needs of loving care, dependence on the mother, and fusional nostalgia are perverted in regression and sadomasochistic degradation. Autistic and stereotypical behaviours display the perversion of the need of autonomy and individuation.

The inpatients find themselves in a terrible isolation: they are separated from all others and, at the same time, a few are individuated, showing a dramatically frail and precarious identity (Di Chiara, 1979).

The alternative is between confusion and anonymity, as the scenes of the women's living quarters and shower rooms show, and brutal isolation, as the scene of the closed dormitories suggest (Figure 5.2).

DOI: 10.4324/9781003381723-5

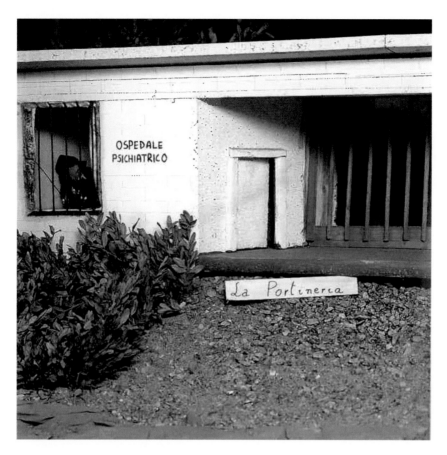

Figure 5.1 The closed entrance gate.

The isolation of the dormitories adds to the social isolation of the asylum and the isolation caused by the closure of the entrance of the ward. This can be interpreted as a scene of sensory deprivation. Sensory experimental deprivation is defined as a condition in which, applying simple devices such as blindfolds, hoods, or earmuffs, some stimuli are reduced or removed from one or more of the senses. In practice, the subject is put in a condition of relative perceptive isolation from the environment. This condition brings forth psychopathological experiences such as space and time disorders, modifications of bodily perception, hallucinations, and other types of confusion. Experimental studies can be correlated to better understand the sensory deprivation caused by congenital or acquired disorders of the sense organs or certain psychiatric pathologies such as schizophrenia and, in particular, the pathology of perceived social isolation. Patients who are already confused are not helped by recognising the

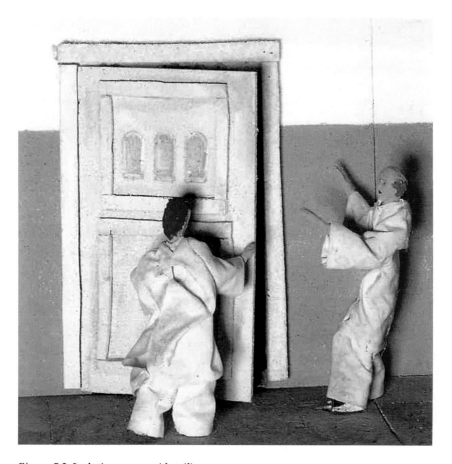

Figure 5.2 Isolation rooms (detail).

differences between internal and external reality and thus reach an adequate level of integration but, on the contrary, the brutality of isolation
forces them to increase and fix their confusion (Petrella, 1969, 1993c).

At first glance, inpatients can be confounded with the plaster of the
wards: they are not only closed in the circumscribed space of the asylum's
walls but are also almost included in the same substance of these walls.
The figures are not distinguishable from the background from which they
should emerge. There is a collusion between their regressive and confusing tendencies and the mimetic tendencies induced from the depersonalising environment. This is because they fear being attacked when
sketches of identity, no matter if normal or pathological but inadequate to
life in the asylum, emerge.

Regression connects the patient to plant life and reduces him to a fossil
resembling something living, a prefiguration of the mortal confusion with

the earth (Pavan and Zappalaglio, 1989). A sleep full of death humiliates and simultaneously protects him.

The scene of the women's living room depicts female patients with various postures and attitudes. It is a lifeless variety from which we cannot glean any meaning because the institutional response denies the possibility of being original and renders everything equal and flat. The woman haranguing the absent-minded crowds and making show of her manic behaviours through her grotesque and disturbing mask cannot be stopped or contained: she is irresponsibly left alone with her words, which cannot take a relational direction or a hint of sharable meaning.

The so-called crazy people do not ask to be heard, only ignored, rejected, set free. This is because inside the institution, their words, no matter if screamed, written, or expressed in some other form, lose their symbolic value, their very meaning. They do not say anything to one another. At best, the words harden into symptoms, for example, manic graphomania, paranoid protest, obsessive, and mannered stylisation (Conforto, 1996).

A woman on a bench, curled up on herself, representing self-confinement, is neither questioned nor recognised nor seen despite the nurses' continuous visual control, rendering them non-existent in a crystalised autism (Figures 5.3–5.10).

Inside the shower room there is neither intimacy nor privacy (Figure 5.11). The sensation of an indecipherable anonymity cancels such rooted feelings as decency and the often-reviled shame. The naked and undefended bodies are offered to the alien and intrusive glances in an atmosphere characterised by a terrible and arbitrary promiscuity. For Lalla Romano (1995), some moments of privacy are essential. Privacy preserves our identity and responds to our instinctive and defensive sense of decency.

In this situation, there is the phenomenon of the negative hallucination of the patient. After the initial and superficial interest of doctors and nurses, the chronic inpatient literally disappears in dark areas or even blind spots, unexperienced gaps of the institutional space. He is reconsidered only when some of his behaviours appear unusual or resounding (Petrella et al., 1978).

Traditional psychiatry divided patients into bad and restless—who were put away in small bedrooms in special wards—and calm and docile, depending on whether they acted out non-aggressively (Figure 5.12).

It is impossible to consider that the aggressiveness of the patient is never purposeless, but is always directed against someone. It implies the presence of the other as a motivating element or witness.

Not only do staff perceive the aggressive tensions but they also must defend themselves from the risk of identifying with patients and thus directly experience the patients' destructive drives. To avoid this difficult

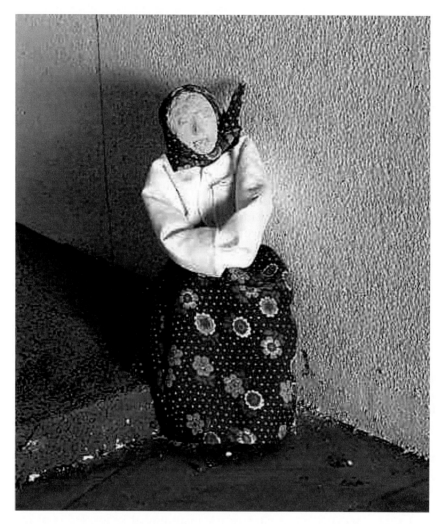

Figure 5.3 Woman in commoner dress in the females' sitting room (detail).

identification, staff can accentuate their professional role and increase and stiffen their distance from patients.

One response to the environmental frustrations is to regress in alienated and passive conduct and in a language without any possibility of symbolisation, the clear expression of a tragic lack of communion. This is a radical renouncement of every kind of affective investment in reality. Another diametrically opposed response is to continuously manifest aggressive conduct, which becomes a crystalised and expensive model of opposing the institutional environment (Petrella, 1993d).

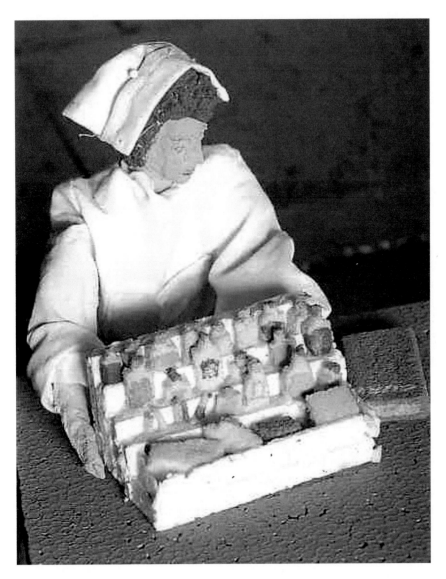

Figure 5.4 Drug distribution in the females' sitting room (detail).

Even the repeated and stereotyped movements of tardive dyskinesia, generally assumed to be a simple neurological syndrome during or after pharmacological treatment for neuroleptics, can be interpreted as attempts of gestural filling and thus a mise-en-scène of the experience of failure. It is a continuous and restless projective activity without which a stable object can be constituted, against which it dies away, or founds a limit (Schinaia et al., 1995).

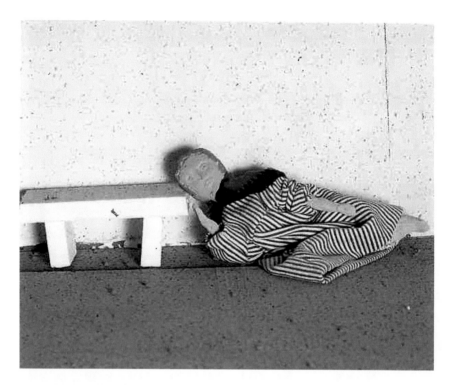

Figure 5.5 Woman lying down a bench in the females' sitting room (detail).

The docile patients take to the extreme the consequences of the institutional aggression because they introject it. They express the experience of institutional aggression through autistic isolation or superficial adaptation to their condition of hospitalised/convict, thus demonstrating collaboration with staff, for example in the maintenance of the ward or assistance of not self-sufficient patients. This is the so-called institutional syndrome clearly described by Erwin Goffman (1961): through identification with the aggressor and by executing nursing-like functions, they deny their sad condition. As Ferenczi says in his seminal "Confusion of Tongues" (1933), in the hope to survive, we sense and "become" precisely what the attacker expects of us—in our behaviours, perceptions, emotions, and thoughts.

The troubled patient tries to become peculiar or a privileged case to save himself from anonymity. Unfortunately, his attempts are doomed to failure not only due to their rigid and de-real character but also because the patient becomes a stereotypical character always playing the same role through which he can act out his impulses in a repetitive and out-of-time dimension.

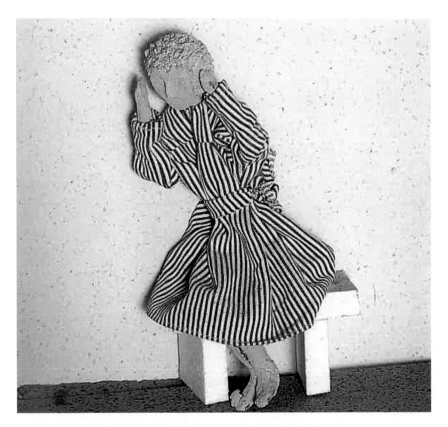

Figure 5.6 Woman with an apron in the females' sitting room (detail).

However patients respond to segregation, as time passes it becomes less valid and efficacious and moves away from the causes that determined it. Thus, this response seems to live in a tragic mechanisation, clearly depicted in the scenes of the crèche.

Petrella (1993a) argues that a locked door is always an objective and impassable barrier. It indicates that we cannot go forward, the path is concretely interrupted, and at best we can continue only through imagination. If a door is the same as a wall, there is a disturbance in communication, a distortion of the meaning of the spaces and uses, a semantic ambiguity that can assume negative and destructive unsuspected values. Of course, to open a door is to remove a material element of constriction, creating the premise for free movement but not concretely achieving it.

After a door opens, there must follow an anti-institutional attitude aiming to also keep open the invisible doors of prejudice, incommunicability, and illiberal constriction. It is necessary to investigate the complex and

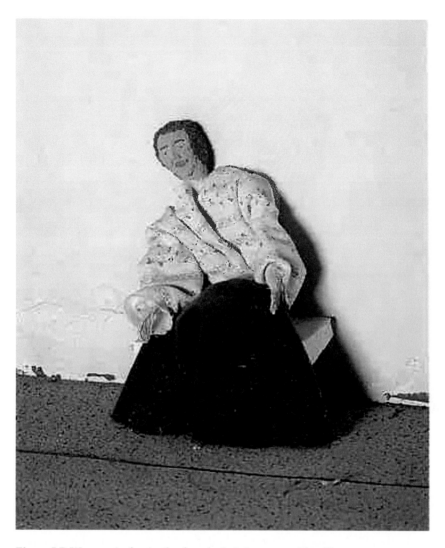

Figure 5.7 Woman in fur in the females' sitting room (detail).

articulated tangle of biological needs and symbolic functions determining a certain disposition and utilisation of the spaces. This investigation allows one to study the preferential routes to where to stay, both entering and exiting, the meeting places, the abandoned and not emotionally invested territories. It is possible to create a map that could represent and reduce communicative and relational obstacles.

Modifying the relational field with our presence, challenging ancient and rooted equilibriums, reviving lost and censored communicative

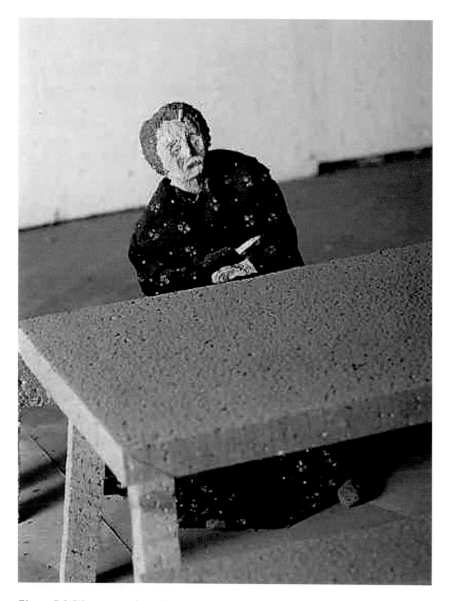

Figure 5.8 Woman at the table in the females' sitting room (detail).

potentials allow one to break the immobility, activation, and movement of fantasies (Ciancaglini et al., 1989).

The closed space of a total institution is the failure of the idea of space as creation, of creating freedom; basically, it is a crossed but not really lived space (Scala, 1975).

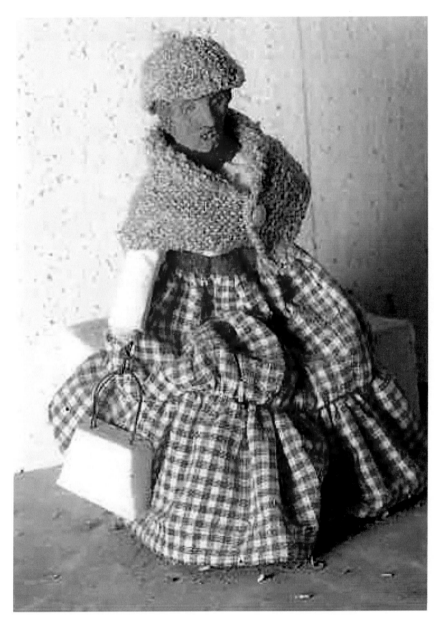

Figure 5.9 Elegant woman in the females' sitting room (detail).

To meet in a communicative space, in which to participate in a common form of life, without becoming lost in a meaningless void, in fragmentation and anxiety, it is not sufficient to spend time with other people and simply sediment the experience of staying together a long

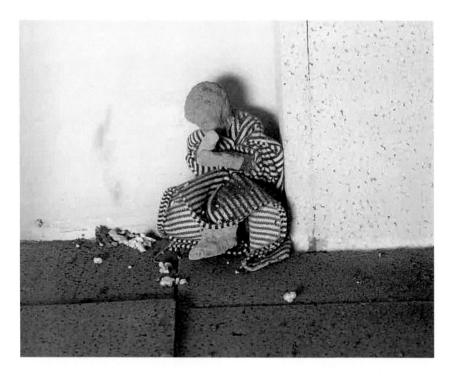

Figure 5.10 Woman sitting on the ground (detail).

time. It is fundamental to have a presence that does not look away, a capacity to understand each other and intrepidly elaborate, and the possibility to develop pleasure and consent—the consent that had always been denied or refused to the psychotic person or deteriorated early on for many different reasons.

Segregation cannot be masked or denied through paternalistic operations as stressed in the scene of the crèche representing a party in a ward during the 1960s (Figures 5.13–5.14).

The sadly feeble lights, the absent looks, and the mechanical moves of the dancers: this scene reveals the deceit and denounces the impossibility of a happiness without freedom. An atmosphere of solitude and alienation covers the couples dancing without enthusiasm, vitality, or rhythm. The dancers look like spectral marionettes confined in isolation and incommunicability. They appear to be forced to have fun only because this is established by the institutional time, of which they are expropriated. The time is articulated from a sort of imperative and external schedule: other people have chronological power they use to decide even the most minute manifestations and expression (De Vincentiis, 1979). The festoons and decorations do not rid the ballroom of its intense squalor:

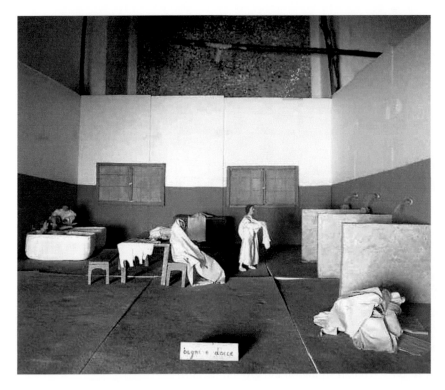

Figure 5.11 Toilets and showers.

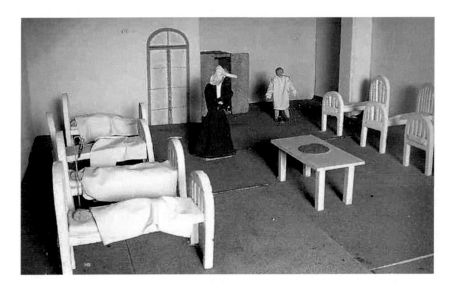

Figure 5.12 The ward's infirmary and the nun.

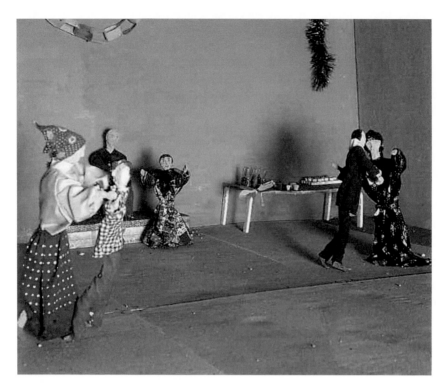

Figure 5.13 The party in the asylum (detail).

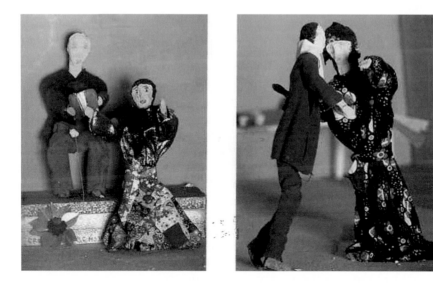

Figure 5.14 The party oin the asylum (details).

indeed, they magnify it and serve as a denunciation of the deceptive machine that is the asylum.

It is historically known that parties had been organised in the asylums since the 19th century. A document found by Manuele Bellonzi (2016) in the National Archive of Florence describes a party in the asylum of Bonifazio: *Domani sera si terrà la festa da ballo autorizzata per il divertimento dei reclusi in manicomio, che comincerà alle 17 e si protrarrà fino alle 23, avendo così deciso il Direttore.*[1] A note of the day after reports: *Nella festa serale non vi è stato alcun inconveniente. Vi hanno partecipato 51 alienati (31 donne e 20 uomini).*[2] The Mad Women's Ball (2019), a María Victoria Mas novel, is about a dance party in 1885. The party was organised in the Salpêtrière Hospital whose head was Charcot: only for a night, the doors of the asylum were opened and the patients, all dressed in elegant vintage clothes, were objects of amusement for the upper middle class.

A party is a moment with many friends, in which isolation is not allowed and everyone can breathe the air of freedom. When the physical and mental spaces are closed, when enthusiasm and emotional engagement are absent, the party becomes a shabby and disrespectful parody. In his book *Il Mio Manicomio* (My Asylum) (2007), Paolo Teobaldi writes that a nurse remembers that, during the parties in the asylum, despite the masks, the gazes of the doctors and nuns were always controlling so that the atmosphere was tense and menacing.

The party in the institution has no carnivalesque transgression, no desperate and limitless collective joy that, at least for a single day, puts power in check.

Freud writes: *A festival is a permitted, or rather an obligatory, excess, a solemn breach of a prohibition. It is not that men commit the excesses because they are feeling happy as a result of some injunction they have received. It is rather that excess is of the essence of a festival; the festive feeling is produced by the liberty to do what is as a rule prohibited* (1913, p. 140).

The party scene of the Nativity at Cogoleto allows observers to feel the rigid and conformist fiction of sociality, the repetitive space, and the uniformed temporality and thus to denounce and unmask these issues much more than a pamphlet or book ever could.

Some segregation aspects (not as tragically explicit as in the scenes of the crèche of Cogoleto) can be found in new psychiatric structures, in the departments dedicated to the care of acute patients and in the territorial mental health services.

Anti-entropic attention must be paid to the counter-transferal defensive attitudes of the health-care workers and the way in which they represent to themselves the assistance and care spaces, lest the old conceptions of "asylum" are surreptitiously restored in a new form, one that is perhaps less evident but nonetheless very dangerous.

Notes

1 "Tomorrow evening a dance party will take place. It was authorised for the amusement of the inmates of the asylum. It will start at 5 p.m. and continue until 11 p.m., as the Head of the Asylum decided."
2 "During the evening party no inconvenience occurred. 51 insane people participated (31 women and 20 men)."

6   The Square

The square is one of the most peculiar architectural spaces of the asylum. Its meaning goes beyond formal implications: it is a representative document of the atmosphere of a historical era.

The square is a big yard on the opposite side of the main gate (Figures 6.1–6.3). It is accessed from the living room, of which it is a sort of natural extension when the weather is good, or the forced alternative when it is time to clean the interiors. The square is a very wide space, in which sometimes trees and flowerbeds can be found, along with benches, tables, and stinking outdoor toilets. It is surrounded by a high metal fence preventing direct contact with the street.

The visitor can easily notice the patients—their faces burned by the sun, their fingers burned by cigarettes—lying on the ground or the bleached benches, or with their noses pressed against the railings watching with astonished grimaces, silent or plaintive, the passers-by beyond the rusty fence.

At least one of the shift nurses stays in the square, in a strategic position, paying attention that no patient can escape from their sight. Staying in the square is a precise task of the nurse, who must preside over that portion of the outdoor area from which the most can be surveilled. The inside-outside opposition permits to spatially distribute other oppositions: organised-disorganised, cosmos-chaos, us-them, and, of course, sane-insane (Petrella, 1993a).

Normally, closed and open are the two poles of a spatial and psychological series going from the home to the street and from the street to the square, through a potentially infinite series of possibilities and combinations. But at the asylum's square this series does not exist. They are denied because there is no gradient and no possible progression from closed to closed.

The presence of a door allowing one to go outside, to an open space, or of a window from which to watch without the limiting mediation of a grid, gives the space a direction, a goal, and thus creates possible alternatives. A door that is always closed contradicts its aim, so a square without freedom is an expression of a regimen giving the space a peculiar

DOI: 10.4324/9781003381723-6

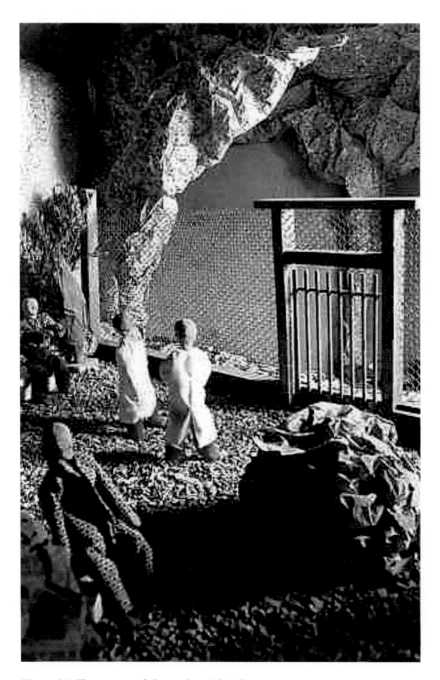

Figure 6.1 The square of the asylum (detail).

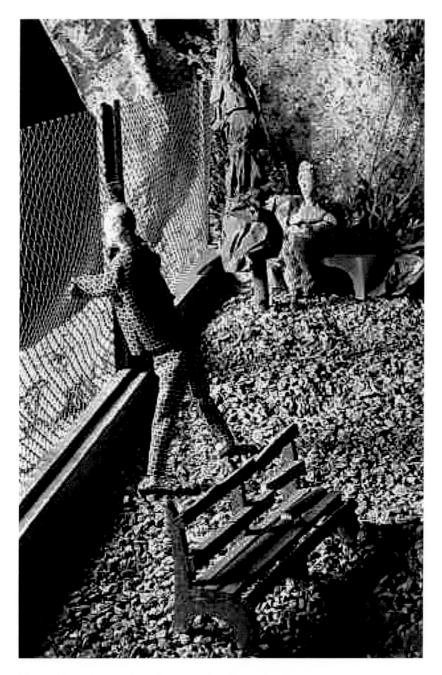

Figure 6.2 Patient against the square's railing (detail).

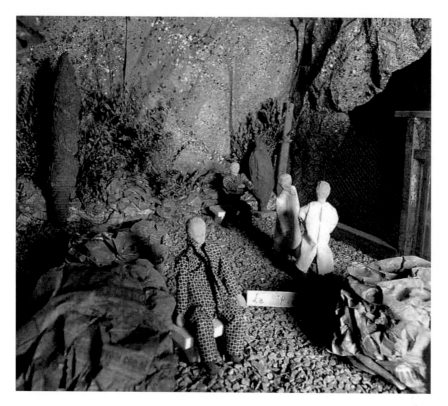

Figure 6.3 Nurses watching over the patients in the asylum's square (detail).

ambiguity. In fact, it is a space that, on the one hand, invites one to act but, on the other, makes the action impossible (Racamier, 1970).

The impossibility of thinking to a passage leads to fantasies about being fused with the mother again and, therefore, to a regression, a false protection against the anxiety of the open spaces or agoraphobic experiences.

Daniel Stern (1985) defines "interpersonal space" as the respect area existing around every human being, no matter child or adult. Its existence is genetically predisposed, the tools for its realisation are innate, but the realisation itself depends on the chance to establish a relationship. The conclusive result of the processes leading to form this "interpersonal space" is fundamental to guarantee a relationship without a prejudice of intrusion and a capacity to feel intimacy, affectivity, and emotional exchanges. The pathologies related to such a space are evident in those clinical cases with defensive rigidity and lack of interpersonal space, when the feeling of an immediate flood occurs on the occasion of a communication coming from the other (Di Chiara, 1994).

Spatial impoverishment can be found in patients who hold catatonic postures that last a long time and look like the foetal position. It seems impossible for them to live in an outside space that is delimited by the perimeter of their body. Space is reduced to a postural bodily experience that genetically comes before the constitution of the object and that pushes away (and sometimes abolishes) every threat and attack coming from the surrounding space (Petrella, 1993a).

At the centre of the *agora* in Ancient Greece, there was the money dealer: it was mandatory to go outside, to an open space, to get currency to make a voyage. The act of coming out alludes to and preludes a detachment from the protection of the motherland. In a condition with a relative absence of points of references, when the risky ghost of a painful experience of bewilderment and insecurity is approaching, the rite proposes to the traveller someone in whom to identify, someone inspiring the capacity of being able to adapt to a new reality, and acquiring new perspectives purified from the most threatening features. The position of the money dealer, at the centre of the city and the square, is umbilical because he deals with the future separation, but it is also a testimony of the collective interest of all the other citizens about those maturational experiences of exploration and return of one of them (Pavan, 1984).

Normally the square grounds inhabitants to everyday life and is simultaneously a landing and passage bridge allowing the citizens to be touched by different forms of life (Isnenghi, 1994). The square is the place of glances, the place in which, more than anywhere else, we can observe each other; here the presence of the others is stopped in our memory; here the snapshot turns into a pose (Pisani, 1990).

In a different manner, the strategical position of the nurse in the middle of the asylum's square cannot be reached. The controlling and controlled gazes do not meet each other; they never touch; there is only a continuous bounce, as in an endless game, of mutual aggressive fantasies occurring in the visual inspection of one of them. Without the continuous visual control of the nurses, the ghost of danger would immediately storm, and, as a result, the patients could be hurt, hurt others, be killed, kill. The response of the patients to this control is the passive renunciation of a contact perceived as painfully violent.

The patient who is always looked at and in the psychotic experience feels the looming gaze of others with anguish, risks feeling overwhelmed and overpowered. The watchman who avoids an encounter that would allow him to penetrate the patient's physiognomy and grasp their essence keeps a distance, objectifies, and reifies the patient. In trying to keep himself distinct, he renounces understanding the other and meeting their gaze. The gaze of the watchman, being only a form of negative self-limitation, promotes in the patient the stiffening in being looked at, in being caught in her or his essence (Sediari et al., 1966).

We know that historically the ancient *agora* was renewed in the Roman forum that was surrounded by a continuous portico unifying the distribution of the road accesses and the entrances to the buildings around it. In turn, it was considered the original matrix of the different types of square (Mancuso, 1971). Entering the forum meant entering a protected space, a container, in which anyone could be a citizen and a charitable person, have conversations and conduct business, meet other people and show himself. It was a truly outdoor theatre in which people were at the same time actors and spectators of collective life.

The medieval square is based on the idea of the Roman forum. In the medieval landscape the theatre does not exist as a building: it occurs in the square. It differs from the forum: the main functions are distributed in various squares, not only in a single place. Here are the council square, the cathedral square, and the market square, often contiguous to each other. The council square represents power, distance, in rigorous geometries: in the Renaissance it became even wider and more geometric, as represented in the "Veduta della Città Ideale" in Urbino.[1] The cathedral square is a sort of neutral field, allowing interactions between the rich and the poor, a meeting forbidden in other areas of the city. The market square is characterised by the colour of the masses and the plebeian crowds engaged in their trades and struggling for survival (Isnenghi, 1994). The asylum's square is neither characterised by the austerity of the council square, nor by the rituality of the cathedral square, nor by the noisy and coloured features of the market square. It is not a place for conversation, social exchanges, or feasts; it is not a container of human histories.

The Renaissance and Baroque squares overwhelmed the historical fabrics and produced a reduction of the city to its representative spaces. During these eras, the concept of square extended itself and included all the urban features whose main purpose was to exalt the monuments and the empty space completely planned, symmetrical, and, therefore, substantially static (Guidoni, 1993).

The squares built in Napoleonic Europe do not communicate with the surrounding buildings and are no longer closed and protected from spatial invasions. They are celebratory places occasionally used for military demonstrations or rallies, generally placed in straight lines, unable to offer stimuli or reasons for spontaneous aggregation moments in the daily life. The role of representation of the squares is re-proposed in moments of concentration of power: in the previous century in Soviet Russia, Nazi Germany, and Fascist Italy.

The celebration of mechanisation and the power of the automobile of some writers (Fitzgerald), artists (Boccioni), and architects (Le Corbusier) indicate that there is no need of the old values of the square anymore (Menozzi, 1993).

Franco Rella (in Cervellini, 1993) argues that the condition in which an individual is immersed today in metropolitan modernity fragments the collective experience of the city and leads to an increasing fragmentation of the collective space of the metropolis.

The square begins to not represent the institutional expression of the identity of the Western cities. Today it is not a viable reality but the metaphor of an absence; it is an ambiguous metaphor between the nostalgia of past and extinct forms of societies (such as the Greek polis) and the desire for a social contract that remains culturally undefined (Balbo, 1993).

The functional decline of the square occurs through the substitution of monuments with bollards and its transformation into a car park. The square as a place of communication disappears when it dissolves into a big service area, in which everything is too large and without proportions, neither for the buildings nor the passers-by (Isnenghi, 1994).

In the asylum there is the extreme destruction of the square, something shaking its conceptual foundations. Here the square is a bleak and grey area, shapeless and sun-drenched, in which identical-looking human beings move slowly, often in puppet-like motion, in solitude, disorderly, without a purpose. They have neither past nor future. Where they come from and where they go is not known.

The scene represents the nurses in uniform, on their own, clearly separated, as if they senselessly controlled the senseless traffic.

Here the space is felt as unbridgeable; it distances, rejects, and prevents any approach or relationship.

The more the square has passed through time and reaches us from very far away, the less likely it presents itself in stylistically pure forms: rather, it bears the traces of all the historical times it has lived through and that lived it.

By contrast, the asylum's square is always the same: a desolate space devoid of both time and history, never tainted or corrupted by the life lived within. It remains a squalid and imperishable monument to the lack of communication.

In his paintings, Giorgio De Chirico represents the square as an enigmatic void: an immense space abandoned by the living, in which buildings and machines appear to live autonomously, regardless of the existence of humans and the utility they and machines can have. Solitude and immobility are at the core of the mystery of paintings about squares in mental asylums.

The square in the Nativity Scene of the Cogoleto asylum refers to the metaphysical intuitions of De Chirico, but with a crucial difference: here the machines are the timeless and lifeless human beings of the asylum, fixed in their lack of words or authentic movements.

This square aims at making its viewer feel death so as to simultaneously give meaning to the end and invite life.

The last projects of transformation of the former psychiatric hospital envisage the demolition of the remaining metal nets and the abolition of these non-squares to build a community centre in the middle of the village-hospital, with a large green area in the front. This area would be the real square, with its umbrellas, passers-by, visitors, businesspeople, charlatans, street artists, acrobats, and musicians. Modifying the model of the square attributes different functions to spaces that are consumed by habit and decay. This change ignites a spark that allows us to better see things, that is, to see them in a new light.

The need for a space used for something that it is not only functional or useful, an area to give room to fantasy, is not only a prerequisite for the individual's mental balance, but it is also one of the fundamental elements for the improvement or decay of group communication. It is an existential need for all the inpatients and hospital workers.

The square would be the place for board games and work, for leisure, power, and people, conflict, and memory.

The community centre becomes a sort of re-invented cafeteria, a part of the diversified architecture of the square. In cafeterias, literature and history have been made, adulteries and revolutions have been committed, journals have been prepared, sonnets and manifestos have been written (Isnenghi, 1994). Perhaps no place shows so suggestive and peculiar an intersection between the private and public as the cafeteria. Cafeterias are hospices for people with broken hearts, and their owners are benefactors offering them a shelter from the storm, like the founders of asylum for the homeless (Magris, 1997).

The community centre can be also a tavern that goes from the periphery to the city centre, to be the place of a sort of socialising, that is more immediate and popular than a snobbish cafeteria. Here we can find not only Campari, slush, hot chocolate, and policy discussions but also a large glass of wine, some focaccia, an obscene joke, and the Gazzetta dello Sport, Italy's most widely read daily newspaper.

The tavern and the church are the two main locales of any self-respecting settlement, two similar places, open to the traveller who wants to rest in the shade in front of a glass of wine. They are two liberal places, in which those who enter are not asked where they come from and under which flag or badge they are (Magris, 1997). The tavern and the church are two typical places of the culture of the square; they are their lasting constitutive elements.

The idea here is to return to the patients meaningful and barrierless places going from their closed-off rooms to the openness of the square. The main aim is to re-introduce socialising as it was in their original culture, in their existential circuit, without any ideological forcing.

In this way, the new square-community centre becomes a central space full of symbolic qualities, an area attracting public and social activities, a confluence of paths. It is plausible to conceive them as symbols of the most extrinsic archetypical elements of a concept of square literally taken from the premodern tradition (Cervellini, 1993). Rather, it is the introduction of a mental-spatial device in complete harmony with the needs of the in-patients, needs that are as formally unexpressed as objectively identifiable.

Aristotle said that all the principles of urbanistic art can be synthesised in the idea that a city must offer safety and happiness at the same time. Perhaps the plan of the community centre cannot offer happiness, but there is a good possibility that it can deliver freedom and socialisation.

Italo Calvino (1983, p. 49) writes: *Squares, streets, flat spaces are open in front of me and displaying an apparent accessibility, as if they say: please, go through us, we are smooth and clear.*

Note

1 "View of the Ideal City," tempera painting, anonymous, 67.5 × 239.5cm, circa between 1470 and 1490. It is in the National Gallery of the Marche, Urbino.

7   The Doctors' Office

If contact with physical disease causes suffering, the relationship with a psychotic patient causes mental anxiety and pain. The counter-transferal defensive movements of staff and the institutional defenses, when in normal conditions, regulate this relationship to avoid identifications that are too painful, which could make therapy and assistance impossible. Unfortunately, when the personal and institutional defensive systems become rigid, they are doomed to failure and transform into symptoms and pathogenic defenses.

The presence of institutional spaces for staff only can sometimes represent a chance of necessary temporary departure from the spaces of madness. However, these spaces must not give the idea of a neat and definitive separation or be a sort of prelude to exclusion and segregation.

The use of technology and drugs can provide a valid support to the relationship and cure if this does not become a technicality or form of interventionism leading to excessive and aggressive treatments.

The use of psychiatric culture, if relativised and considered in a wide relational and social context, can be meaningful, if compiling medical records, writing anamneses, and making diagnoses and prognoses do not become objectifying operations, unable of stressing the emotional substance of the relationship.

In psychiatric hospitals, defensive mechanisms to protect from uncomfortably close contact with madness are sometimes obvious and flagrant, sometimes hidden and subtle. In general, health-care workers are not aware of the relationship between these mechanisms and the anxiety caused by the encounter with mental suffering and tend to rationally explain behaviours that are illogical and self-defeating. The most manifest among the institutional defenses is the neat separation of the rooms for staff and those for patients. Staff occupy patient areas only to clean and try to cure; a moment more than necessary can be too risky and dangerous and lead to psychic contagion.

Doctors tend to stay closed in their rooms to protect and reinforce their identity, which is hard-tested by their meetings with patients; nurses, who

DOI: 10.4324/9781003381723-7

are forced to be exposed to patients for longer periods, use more direct and more authoritative ways to avoid spending time with them.

The nurses' changing rooms are not on the same floor as the hospitalisation area, just as there are different kitchen, toilets, and common areas for staff. Locked doors that only staff can open highlight this difference and the fact that there are areas that are forbidden to patients.

The division of spaces inside the asylum is not a degeneration of the original project that was favourable for patients at the start. On the contrary, from the beginning, the officially declared purpose was evaded, just before the asylum was active and operative (Saraceno, 1982). The fear of close contact and its attendant mental contagion, strictly connected to fantasies about touching dirt and contracting infective diseases, justify the use of segregation's measures (Petrella, 1993e).

Even today we can find some rites, such as cleaning the keys with soap and water many times a day, accentuating the fear of contamination, a fear so strong as to prevail over the well-rooted sense of decency. Until recently, when female nurses left the hospitalisation spaces and entered the kitchen, they took off their uniforms.

The defensive mechanisms of the doctors are less explicit but no less strong and meaningful. Their time with patients is minimal and mostly dedicated to routine administrative issues.

Psychiatrists rarely entered the hospitalisation areas, which are generally locked. They received in their office patients who needed to be cured or whose behaviour they must assess in order to maintain order in the ward. In such a case, two nurses took the patient to the doctor's room, reported the patient's condition to the doctor, and protected the doctor from possible injuries, whose scary ghost inexorably hovered.

If the door of the doctor's room is left open longer than usual, it does not mean that the room is accessible. Rather, it can be even more inaccessible than that of the nurses' room because of a demarcation line that is as invisible as it is strongly interiorised.

As represented in a scene (Figure 7.1), the doctors in their white coats are behind closed doors, safely shut away in their rooms, where they speak between amongst themselves so as to avoid bearing witness to the mental pain of the patient and any subsequent threats to their identity. Their rooms are far from the wards, so they maintain (or, perhaps more accurately, believe to maintain) contact with the patient *in effigie*, by looking at their photograph on the title page of the patient medical record. In this manner, they construct an unanimated and unneedy puppet in place of the real patient.

There is a photograph so that staff can identify a particular patient amongst the many patients the overcrowded wards. It was taken when the patient entered the asylum, when the strong use of institutional therapies had not yet changed their facial expression. Had been taken later, the patient's face would have appeared so inexpressive and

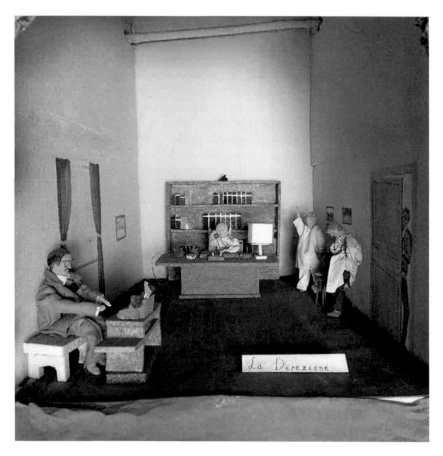

Figure 7.1 The doctors' office (detail).

anonymous as to render it difficult to identify its possessor. The diagnostic use of photography is based on the predominant role of the physiognomic in the anthropological sciences during an era when the domain of the gaze was undisputable. Photography in psychiatry aims to put distance between the psychiatrist and their object of inquiry and defend the psychiatrist from mental pain. The relationship between the patient in the photograph on the medical record permits the psychiatrist to eliminate all relational distortions and offer a directly observable image of cleanliness typical of a certain positivism (Schinaia, 2001, 2004, 2005).

The photograph gives its user the pleasure of being a safe spectator. What is monstrous can be shown and observed in a phalanstery or panopticon in which the descriptive narrative mediates all the anxieties of contact (Zappalaglio and Pavan, 1986).

The photograph takes the subject away from their original human context and every other dimension, save for the pathological one, that can be seen in their disturbed mimicry, often exaggerated by grimaces.

The deceit of the photograph is to diminish the extent of subjective distortions by fixing the fleeting observation and permitting the patient to repeat it when necessary. The coefficient of deception is bigger because a photograph, as well as every form of recording, has the inconvenience of making appear possible what is false (Bion, 1962). But the photograph of the clinical record could give to the observer an image of the person of many years ago, which can tell the history of the women and men photographed and their anxieties. Cowherds, professors, office employees, and factory workers are recognisable by the hem of their collarless shirts, their soft or rigid collars, their haircuts, and their lapels. The smiling face of the mentally retarded who comes from the countryside can be a sign of an accepted and shared disability is opposed to the smiling (but slightly scared and astonished) face of the mentally retarded who comes from the city, probably more isolated in their family, certainly more blamed. Austere or scruffy haircuts can frame the sad faces of depressed widows, be they wealthy bourgeoises consumed by grief or housewives with many children to feed, whose faces are passively hardened by the loss of the sole provider for the family. The social contexts, living spaces, and geographical environments are never the background of these apparently timeless faces. It is nonetheless possible to appreciate the variety of expressions that can be attentive, curious, careless, uninterested, cheerful, relaxed, sad, rough, open, moved, closed, fixed, understandable, and unfathomable. However, both the proxemics and the phantasy can help us to reconstruct, imagine, guess, and discover an absolutely original internal world and an unexplored relational possibility, which must find a representation for the construction of such a scenography of the meeting (Schinaia et al., 1992).

The medical record itself is a cold and anonymous logbook in which the biographical and environmental notes of the patient, the description of their symptoms, the date of meetings and visits, and the pharmacological prescriptions are reported. It does not contain the emotional richness of encounters with the patient, the development of their history, the struggles of the therapist, the contacts with the environment, the hermeneutic attempts to understand; rather, it contains boring lists of events without semantical or syntactical aim, written in a technical and scientific language that serves mainly to defend and add distance. It is a language that does not say much, allow a narrative, or invent and tell stories, the possible myths for the patient (Schinaia and Soldi, 1985).

Freud (1893) writes about his experience at Pitié-Salpêtrière Hospital in Paris and describes Jean-Martin Charcot as a dominant force naming the animals in a zoo or the plants in a botanical garden. He reminds him of

Adam, whom God instructed to distinguish every living being in the Garden of Eden and give it a name.

This is how Jung (1989, p. 114) describes his experience at Burghölzli, the psychiatric hospital in Zürich, directed by Eugen Bleuler: *Psychiatry teachers were not interested in what the patient had to say, but rather in how to make a diagnosis or how to describe symptoms and to compile statistics. From the clinical point of view which then prevailed, the human personality of the patient, his individuality, did not matter at all.*

A medical record aiming to provide a hyper-detailed image of the patient is like the paradox of the cartographers of the Emperor of China as told by Borges and Bioy Casares (1967). They were asked to draw a map of the Empire as precisely and correctly as possible and thus, after many attempts, created a map as big as the Empire itself that the next generations cruelly dismissed leaving it to the effects of the Sun and the Winter.

The traditional medical record looks like the *bourrage*, an ancient psychiatric term referring to the graphical productions of certain institutionalised psychotics filling many sheets of paper with a lot of words and signs. From these sheets it is impossible to define a global and coherent image, but what is clear is the underlying *horror vacui*.

The history emerging from the record of the anamnestic data is a text without the features of time and identity: it does not have the features of a "tissue" in which generativity and creativity should stay (Barthes, 1973).

Every communication is reduced to the passive adjustment to a pseudoscientific institutional language having the illusory necessity to be comprehensible to everyone who wants to check the record. In this sense, there is the contradiction between the presence of a unique and unrepeatable text and that of a generic and massifying language. However, even in that arid language there are signs of emotional communication, for example in the form of errors revealing the presence of a humanity. Writing a history in a medical record cannot be a neutral event: it is always a more or less voluntary translation of the text about the world of the patient.

The incorrect usage of a participle or other verbs, the presence of a neologism with vague dialectal sounds, the omission of a word that simultaneously renders the text incomprehensible and opens it to different interpretations like an ambivalent message of the Pythia, the priestess of the Temple of Delphi relaying the response of Apollo: a Mario becoming a Maria or, more generally, a lag or a stop or a caesura or an acceleration of the syntactic rhythm, can shed light on the pieces of an unreported history [*saxa loquuntur* Freud (1907) reported at the start of the Gradiva], on the feelings of the person who compiled the record that did not materialise in a written form but are waiting to be unveiled by a non-preconceived examination that goes beyond words (Schinaia et al., 1994).

Institutional work demands that we look through these photographs and histories for more open developments and futures (and thus not fatalistically biased by a continuous prejudice). But looking through them cannot be done in the closed and set-apart doctors' rooms: it must be a fundamental part of the therapeutic relationship. This necessitates remaining at the heart of institutional reality, in the hospitalisation areas, in the places of socialisation, in which the Other is a flesh and blood human being to meet, not a number or medical record.

8   Electroshock

Electroshock, also known as electroconvulsive therapy or ECT, was created in 1938. It was discovered randomly, not as part of a psychiatric research project. The Italian neuro-psychiatrist Ugo Cerletti was the Director of Anatomic-Pathology at the Psychiatric Hospital of Milan and was working on finding a way to artificially provoke seizures to test on dogs and rats changes in the *Cornu Ammonis* areas of the hippocampus. When he was Director of the University Clinic in Rome, he observed that a 125-volt current produced seizures in pigs. If they were not slaughtered, they awoke without showing any apparent damage (Cerletti and Bini, 1938).

Cerletti (1950) described the first patient subjected to ECT, a schizophrenic in his 40s, as a someone who expressed himself exclusively in incomprehensible gibberish made up of odd neologisms and whose identity was unknown since he arrived from Milan by train without a ticket. Cerletti administered the first ECT on a human as he and his then assistant Lucio Bini had done with dogs, by affixing two electrodes soaked in salt solution to the patient's temples with an elastic band and, as a precaution for the first test, reducing the current (70-volt) and duration (0.2 seconds). He reported that the patient suddenly jumped on his bed and tensed of all his muscles. Then, he immediately collapsed on the bed without losing consciousness and started to sing at the top of his lung. Finally, he fell silent. Cerletti concluded that this test showed evidence that, based on the previous experiments with dogs, the voltage had been too low. Cerletti and Bini discussed whether they should administer another electric shock with higher voltage. As they were debating this, the patient said, in a comprehensible language, "Not a second. Deadly." Against the opinion of the majority, Cerletti decided on a second shock.

He reapplied the electrodes on the patient's head and administered a 110-volt current for 0.5 seconds. Again the patient immediately and briefly cramped of all his muscles. After a brief pause, a typical epileptic fit occurred. Everyone was impressed during the patient's tonic phase with apnoea, ashy paleness, and cadaverous facial cyanosis. The apnoea seemed painful and endless, contrary to how it is when it occurs

DOI: 10.4324/9781003381723-8

spontaneously. The bystanders anxiously stood by until the first deep and stertorous inhalation and shudders. Finally, to everybody's immense relief, the patient demonstrated a typical gradual awakening. He sat up without any help, appeared calm, and vaguely smiled, as if he were expecting a question. Cerletti asked him what had happened to him, and he answered without gibberish that he did not know, perhaps he had fallen asleep. This is the origin of electroshock and the reason why it was named in this way.

Cerletti hypothesised that the artificial seizures the electric current provoked in the brain could have acted as antagonists of schizophrenia, assuming that the epileptic seizure and the schizophrenic manifestation were mutually incompatible. The idea of curing a disease by provoking another was not new: in the 1920s the Austrian Nobel Prize winner Wagner von Jauregg treated progressive paralysis by inoculating malaria. Manfred Sakel used this method and, for the first time, developed insulin shock therapy to treat schizophrenia.

Ladislas J. Meduna introduced the antagonism between epilepsy and schizophrenia with Cardiazol shock therapy, and in 1938, Cerletti based his ideas on Meduna's studies (Balduzzi, 1962).

Although the discovery of electroshock occurred in the electro-physiological realm, its introduction radically altered Italian asylums. In the 1940s, these asylums mainly used seaweed therapy, which consisted of throwing the agitated patient naked in a cell covered with litter sprinkled with dried seaweed. This occurred after the Second World War because electroshock, after being discovered in Italy, was immediately exported to the United States where it was widely used, especially with the soldiers fighting at the war front.

Freud (1920a, p. 216) passed negative judgement on the use of ECT in treating war trauma: *Since his illness (war neurosis) served the purpose of withdrawing him from an intolerable situation, the roots of illness would clearly be undermined if it was made even more intolerable to him than active service. Just as he had fled from the war into illness, means were now adopted which compelled him to flee back from illness into health, that is to say, into fitness for active service. For this purpose, painful electrical treatment was employed, and with success.*

Although it was discovered in Italy, electroshock as a psychiatric technique was imported from the United States. This violent and empirical treatment for the first time forced the physician to create a relationship with the psychiatric patient that, up until then, was inexistent. However, when time revealed that the core of schizophrenia could not be attacked with convulsive shocks, scientific ideology took two distinct and alternative paths: obsessive technicism and the disintegration of the patient (Balduzzi, 1969). The first changes of modified Cerletti's primitive method were Tierz's low-voltage glissando shock, rectified-current electroshock, pulse electroshock, square-current, greek-current, compound-current, and "wave and spike" electroshocks.

The most important modification was ECT protected with succinyl-choline, an anaesthetic that on the one hand eliminated inconveniences such as bone fractures but on the other increased the probability of pro-longed apnoea. At that time many psychiatrists became experts in anaesthesia and reanimation so they could use electroshock and face its collateral effects.

Italian asylums used electroshock less and less partly due to the recognition that it was often prescribed improperly but also because succinylcholine eliminated pain and its underlying features of sadistic-punitive ritual. The amnesic-confusion syndrome following a destructive use of electroshock was considered a therapeutic technique. This was the origin of electroshock annihilation syndrome (Catalano Nobili and Cerquetelli, 1972).

Electroshock was a repressive instrument for a long time: all it took for staff to use it, was an agitated or disobedient patient.

The scene of the crib dedicated to electroshock represents the aura of mystery and terror surrounding this treatment (Figure 8.1). It is a mystery for those who have never been so unlucky as to be treated with such a painful instrument. Terrified is the glance of those who already ex-perienced the passage of current without anaesthesia and are forced for pseudoscientific or disciplinary reasons to feel the pain of applying the electrodes again.

The room of electroshock is characterised by an intense realism: the "magical box" occupies the centre of the space and is accurately re-produced. It clearly shows that aura of suspension and ritual death around the shock experience. It is a sort of *memento mori* with a high deterrent potential towards anyone who wants to define himself through his language and behaviour against the institutional order.

The central position of the electroshock device aims to attribute to the psychiatrist a technological power that makes his task objective, but the presence of four patients lying in bed in the same room highlights the sad routine reality of a serial treatment. The people in the white coats believe that the people in the beds are soulless machines that another machine can repair and put back in the institutional circle as in an assembly line.

The screams of pain and fear coming from that centrally located room, usually very close to the doctors' office, serve as a warning that all must obey the law of arbitrariness and prevarication of man on man.

Thus, punishment and torture were masked by therapeutical needs; it was sadism in the name of science; violence in the name of normality. The little device, which at the beginning of its introduction in the asylum could perhaps allow physicians to approach their patients, seemed as an apparently precise instrument impending any chance of relationship; pain and fear were not the object of the cure, but only the necessary fallout of a therapeutic method.

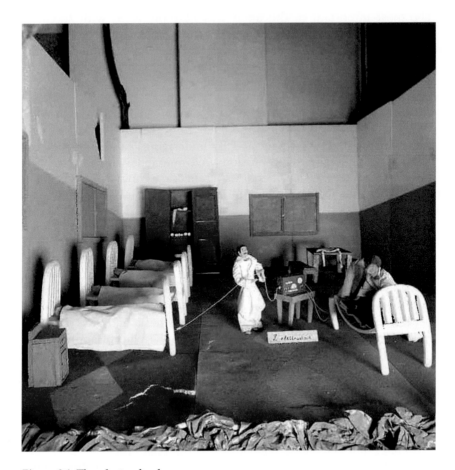

Figure 8.1 The electroshock.

On July 12, 1974, the Head of the Psychiatric Hospital of Collegno in Turin, Giorgio Coda, was found guilty and convicted to five years in prison for abusing patients, banned from public office forever and from the medical profession for five years. In their sentence, the judges argued that transcranial and lumbo-pubic electromassage had punitive, not therapeutic, aims, the treatments were illegitimate, and the hospital was a place of terror psychosis and inhuman and vexatious life regimen (Papuzzi, 1977).

In the first years after its introduction, electroshock therapy was successful because patients tended to respond both to the quantity and quality of attention they received. Psychiatrists had much interest and enthusiasm about this therapy and they were forced to establish at least a minimal relationship with the patient. In other words, the psychiatrist believed that the patient responded only to the electroshock, when the patient also responded to the psychiatrist's enthusiasm for the new treatment. And this enthusiasm was very intense because it promised release from the frustration of dealing with a "refractory disease." In fact, knowing that the agitation of a patient could be calmed thanks to a simple action completely modifies the emotional attitude of the physician. Of course, this is the same for the patient (Racamier, 1970).

Now, in the realm of the psychiatric culture, there are two opposite positions about the use of electroshock, one radically critical, the other thoughtlessly enthusiastic.

In the conference proceedings of the Réseau internazionale di alternativa alla psichiatria (International network for an alternative to psychiatry) (1977), the movement Psichiatria Democratica (Democratic Psychiatry) argues against every kind of shock therapy, even those apparently less damaging versions such as unilateral shock, insulin shock, and acetylcholine shock. These interventions are considered violent and having the only goal to control the patient. They often cause irreversible cerebral and/or bodily damage rather than any therapeutic benefit.

Electroshock is the clearest example of non-participative therapy: there is no free and aware participation on behalf of the patient, only the imposition of silence and oblivion.

Breggin (1979) describes the deceptive ways in which the subjectivity of the patient as a fundamental requirement for the therapy was excluded. The paradox here is the use of electroshock with the implicit aim of the patient's annihilation.

Jervis (1975) strongly argues that using electroshock is like giving a kick to a malfunctioning television. Berke (1972) points out that the physician using electroshock kills the pain but ignores the wound. Sullivan (1940) writes that the philosophy of electroshock can be roughly summarised as that it is better to be a happy imbecile than a schizophrenic.

According to some scientific positions in the psychodynamic tradition, the meaning of electroshock is episodical and ahistorical. It should not be considered a therapeutic process. The time factor, something fundamental in the mental functioning of a person, is completely ignored. The risk is that, after a treatment, the patient does not know how he received electroshock or how he came out of it.

According to the Comitato Nazionale per la Bioetica (Italian Bioethics Committee) (1996), there is the risk of not understanding an implicit message from the patient, who can communicate his "intention" to not look inside himself, to not discuss himself, to not have any confrontation with himself. Asking or "accepting" electroshock is akin to asking for unconsciousness, sleep, death—that is, for the end of everything.

Electroshock stops questions and messages, always devalues every form of listening. It deceptively appears therapeutic, but silences conflicts and contradictions, features of the mind that normally resist to manifest, and fragments the possibility of a subject to be herself or himself and to gain her or his identity (Ferro F.M., 1979).

Crepet and Righetti (1985) stress that this is a historic moment in which biologism returns. Such a biologism is different from that of the past, it does not have any subjective implication, it has been "cleaned up." In such a significant moment, there is the risk of electroshock being seen as an efficacious and useful device, which can be used without any serious implication, especially if it is applied one time. Crepet and Righetti describe an extreme case as much more like a situation induced by an institution than the genuine expression of suffering. They argue that electroshock is not an empirical measure for extreme cases, that is, a device that must be used when nothing else works; rather, it is the repetition of something wrong, in which there cannot be any assessment, relationship, or attribution of meaning.

Along with the supporters of the death of the "magic box," many psychiatrists, generally North American and British, with a neurological-biologistic background, argue that the use of electroshock can be beneficial for the acute psychosis and melancholia. They support their claims with positive statistical data (Royal College of Psychiatrists, 1977; American Psychiatric Association, 1989; 1990; Nolen and Haffmans, 1989; Coffey and Weiner, 1990; Lader and Herrington, 1990; Persad, 1990). Based on such data, in 1996 the Consiglio superiore della sanità (National Institute of Health)-decided to extend the possibility to prescribe electroshock therapy by including disorders such as depression, mania, schizophreniform disorder, schizophrenia, catatonia, neuroleptic malignant syndrome, serious disorders during pregnancy, and puerperal psychosis. The neurobiologistic choices, that now risk being dominant in psychiatry, are more ideological than scientific because they do not consider the great results of the psychiatrists who strongly reduced the use of electroconvulsive therapy. Further, they are ill-conceived by an organicistic prejudice more dangerous than any anti-psychiatric prejudice.

Some psychiatrists argued that electroshock revokes the experience of death and thus can cure the melancholics by fantastically satisfying their need of self-punishment. For (Racamier, 1970), this is unacceptable because it presupposes a confusion between melancholia and masochism.

It is also argued that electroshock can constitute a big and immediate discharge of aggressive or erotic energies, the biological and disorganised prefiguration of a murder or an orgasm (Flesher, 1949). These and other similar considerations clearly show that there is nothing to understand of a method more likely belonging to the magical than the scientific realm.

The book *La Borde ou Le Droit à la Folie* (Polach and Sivadon-Sabourin, 1976) describes awakening after electroshock as a moment of truth than nothing escapes, something absolutely pertaining to the objects, in which there is the rawness of the forms, the depth of music, the mask of a smile. For the authors electroshock is the encrypted response to a symptom; it should be the introduction of a break-up in a chronic depression frustrating everything or in a confusing anxious state; it should bring about the return of some potentialities and, in some cases, their discovery.

This exaggerated generalisation of the outcomes of electroshock therapy shows how a certain psychoanalytic justificationism can be harmful and distort observations that, if relativised, can be meaningful: for example, the value of the symbolic meaning regarding the dramatisation of the realm death-resurrection (Bertolini and Casarino, 1974).

Fenichel (1945) points out that the (conscious or unconscious) attitude of the physicians using electroshock was generally something like "to kill and to revive." He assumes the presence of implicit omnipotent and sadomasochistic phantasms in the ideology of the physicians prescribing and using electroshock.

Physicians often prescribe electroshock therapy not because of the symptoms or the diagnosis but because of an almost always unrecognised tension in the psychiatrist-patient relationship. The psychiatrist tends to find a radical solution to remove this tension.

The impetus that sometimes leads physician to use electroshock can be a signal of countertransference malaise. Thus, it follows that electroshock is a sort of *acting out*, perhaps the most extreme defense from sharing the intolerable suffering of the patient (Breggin and De Girolamo, 1987).

Electroshock permits the psychiatrist to free the patient from his symptoms quite quickly, instead of working with him to find the meaning and nature of the disease and thus to help him to work through the crisis and to deal with the difficult process of facing the suffering, with the hope of gaining an albeit painful recovery. Electroshock would be helpful in fighting the crisis by shortening it, but it would not elaborate it positively.

It is not wise to take part in the sort of war waged between the supporters and opponents of the use of electroshock. It is much better to denounce the ideological conditionings underlying its generalised practice and radical renounce. In some peculiar cases, electroshock could be useful.

The fear of the aggressive and sexual tendencies that electroshock can evoke sometimes leads not to an excess of prescription but to a phobic proscription. It is worth noting that the secondary rationalisations are always at disposal for insufficiently justifying unrealistic positions (Racamier, 1970).

The use of electroshock has been justified in those cases in which there was no chance to make something in the course of those mental diseases leading to death. Nonetheless, there are many doubts about its specific efficacy in the long and short term.

Epidemiological data on electroconvulsive therapy are incomplete and fragmentary but show that most developed countries restrict its use to cases of drug-resistant major depression. On the contrary, in many developing countries it is much more prescribed for a plethora of clinical conditions such as schizophrenia, depression, mania, anorexia nervosa, etc. (De Girolamo, 1993).

Generalising the use of electroshock to all the cases of melancholia appears to be arbitrary and dangerous. However, using it in cases of major depressive disorder with psychomotor inhibition and resistant to high and prolonged use of antidepressants could be useful in reducing mental pain and avoiding death. The formulation of this principle is based on two prescriptions: the first has to do with the caregiver's verification of his own feeling of desperation related to his therapeutic impotence; the second prescription has to do with the verification of the feeling that the patient is in serious and immanent vital risk. Of course, there are some sources of error in applying this principle. But I believe they can be avoided by observing two fundamental rules correcting possible relational distortions: first, never decide alone or only after discussing with those workers directly involved in the case—in other words, decisions should be made after meeting with all the staff and the team and involving members who do not deal with the clinical case; second, do not hurry, take as much time as possible to clarify the opinions and arguments coming from the discussions, possibly after many conversations with the relatives of the patient (Pavan and Schinaia, 1980).

Instead of a militarised scientific position, it is necessary to emphasise only the interests of the suffering person and to completely assume the responsibility of using a risky tool, whose mechanisms of action are still unknown (this point also applies to many drugs), with a negative history, and with temporary but significant collateral effects (memory disorders). It must be assessed if this therapy can soothe mental pain and perhaps even save a life.

The Nativity Scene evokes an aura of suspension and sadism around the rite of passage of the electric current. It warns us against the dangers of abusing or ideologically using this tool. It also reminds us that psychiatry must deal with a flesh and blood person with his passions and pains, not with an inanimate object on which to unemotionally make therapeutic pseudo-experimentations.

In 1995, the Comitato Nazionale per la Bioetica (Italian Bioethics Committee) argued that, at that moment, according to the peculiar ethical relevance of the general principles of informed consent, there were no bioethical reasons to doubt the validity and reliability of electroconvulsive therapy as indicated in scientific literature. In the same document, the Committee invited physicians to use electroshock prudently and after a careful medical examination of every case and an assessment of possible valid and reliable alternatives. Finally, it stressed the ethical necessity of making every effort to obtain informed consent, in spite of the great difficulties to gain it from a psychiatric patient and his representatives.

The physician and his team, with their conscience, knowledge, and ethics, must make a choice in very painful and peculiar cases. It is a choice that recalls fantasies of ritual death but that can lead to life. It must respect the principle that calls for external organisms to apply rigorous control of all these specific and potentially dangerous practices and techniques. In 1997, the Italian Ministry of Health created a committee to work on the use of electroconvulsive therapy. The committee concluded that electroshock can be used only in public or authorised private institutes, with the mandatory presence of a psychiatrist and anaesthetist. Further, it necessitated the clear expression of the patient's free and informed consent. In those cases in which the patient cannot give such consent, electroshock can be administered only in public recovery and cure structures after a clinical report written and signed by at least two psychiatrists attesting to its absolute necessity.

9   The Children's Ward

Dorothy Burlingham and Anna Fredu (1943) observe that in the first two years of the developmental phases of personality the child shows his maturational progresses mainly in the control of muscles and independent motility. They are mainly due to innate and internal causes, not external circumstances. Rather, language, the capacity to feed autonomously, and sphincter control are intrinsically related to the degree of intimacy of the mother-child relationship and constant interaction between maturational forces and external stimuli.

René Spitz (1965) stresses that at the beginning of infancy, the social realm of the child is constituted of the mother mediating all the forces in the environment through her preverbal and emphatic communication and feeding. When this support is missing, as when children are in-stitutionalised early in life, severe distortions or developmental delays can occur. In fact, if in the first year of life children are deprived of all the objectual relations for more than five months, they show an increasingly serious deterioration, which appears to be, albeit partially, irreversible.

Studies on anaclitic depression and severe emotional deprivation dis-order helped to change societal attitudes about hospitalisation in paedi-atric wards. Now, the length of hospitalisation for children is the minimum necessary, and, in all cases, the mother must concretely and stably be there.

For those children displaced from their home during war, Winnicott (1984) recommended preserving their sense of continuity by gathering news, pictures, objects, every kind of memory about their past. In the child, the breaking of continuity can lead to privation and deprivation. For Winnicott (1965) privation is the origin of psychosis: it is the failure of the first basic supports from the environment. The failures of the *holding* function determine the annihilation of the individual, whose existential continuity is interrupted. An alternative situation can occur when en-vironmental supports are initially good but then stop. These supports allow an important degree of organisation of the Ego and then fail at a certain stage, before the individual can create an internal environment,

DOI: 10.4324/9781003381723-9

that is, can become independent. For Winnicott (1984), this deprivation does not cause psychosis but the development of an antisocial tendency.

In the 1950s and 1960s, many studies were conducted on the damage caused by maternal deprivation and the very early removal of children from their families and their consequent institutionalisation.

In the UK, Robertson (1958) started his inquiries on the consequences of infant hospitalisation. He documented his experience in the film *A Two-Year-Old Goes to Hospital*, which drove positive change in the conditions of paediatric wards.

Bowlby (1951) carried out for the WHO (World Health Organization) a research on the psychological conditions of children living far from their families and pointed out that, if a community cares about children, it must take care of their parents.

In the US, Senn and Provence studied the influence of a stay in an institution and healthy practices on infant development (Senn, 1949).

Since the 1940s, five years before Spitz, Bakwin (1942) stressed that children staying in a hospital without their mothers tended to succumb and deteriorate.

Richards (1979), an ethologist who later became Family Research Professor at the University of Cambridge, reviewed the possible effects of separation at the neonatal age. Despite his copious data, his studies and positions were not considered until much later, especially in the psychiatric realm.

Maccacaro (1973) writes that both the psychiatric and the paediatric hospital reduce the patient to an object, deny his identity, history, and social class, and destroy with every weapon and cruelty his subjectivity. In the case of the paediatric hospital, this reduction of the child to an object is practiced by excluding the residual maternal subject from the institution.

In Italy, the situation remained almost the same until the 1960s. During that decade, shelters for infants and special schools with differentiated classrooms proliferated: this clearly confirmed the condition of separation and discrimination of children from their family or peers (Ammaniti, 1995).

In 1970 the total number of institutionalised minors was 400,000, of whom 110,000 were in orphanages. Three-quarters of minors attending special schools did so in a mental institution.

In 1978, the year of the Basaglia Law, the paediatric ward of the Psychiatric Hospital of Cogoleto was still open and active. The mean number of hospitalised children, between the ages of 3 and 13, was around 50, except in the years preceding the closure of the ward, when new admissions were suspended. The older children were transferred to the adult wards and, only in few cases, in new group homes organised for this purpose.

Infamous ward No. 10 was the final receptacle of psychotic, disabled, and traumatised children, whose common mark was their social dangerousness.

In 1944, the psychiatrist and Italian Republic Senator Adriano Ossicini denounced the bad living conditions for the children hospitalised in the psychiatric hospital Santa Maria della Pietà (Our Lady of Sorrows) in Rome. He bemoaned the scientific absurdity of shutting children away in asylums. He also showed that this practice allowed hospitals to be refunded, as the law prescribed. Further, he stressed that even juridically the children were considered as adult sectioned patients. (Ossicini, 1973) points out that concepts such as dangerousness and awkwardness were used generically and without cheques, as well as concepts like possibility or impossibility of rehabilitation. This random and perverse use of these concepts generated confusion because the institutes put together very different subjects, classified as idiots or imbeciles, mentally retarded, mongoloids, people with personality disorders, "abnormal," potential criminals, unstable, a-social, genetically ill-suited for familial, financial, and social matters. These and similar institutes lacked, not only personnel with sufficient expertise in assistance and education, able to establish a personal relationship with the children but also any chance for psychotherapies, not even if there were psychotherapists in these inhuman structures.

Visitors to the wards witnessed something horrifying: children—often weather-beaten and naked or, at best, in ragged clothes—were in rooms reeking of faeces and urine, desolate, devoid of furniture, save for squalid benches pushed against the walls. Some children were in restraints and straitjackets, purportedly to protect them from self-harm but in reality because it made the task of the staff easier. At night, when the number of nurses on shift decreased, the number of restraints on the little patients greatly increased.

Staff concentrated all their efforts on cleaning the ward as much as possible so the children were left alone. They chased each other or moved without any apparent aim: some injured themselves due to the absence of harmony in their movements and the inadequacy of the spaces; some isolated themselves in a corner, often leafing through or tearing up a magazine or scraps of paper, sometimes covering the floor with a carpet of paper; some rhythmically and repeatedly banged their head against the wall.

All the toys in the ward were destroyed because the children could not break the usual schemes of inactivity, autonomously change their aggressive behaviours, and adopt more productive and creative models and forms recalling even a sketch of play. The institution did not propose any detailed didactive attempt. Instead, the nuns confiscated by the toys so they could not be destroyed. The nurses were not only insufficient in number, but they also lacked any qualification in paediatrics and suffered the physical and psychological wear that greatly reduced their ability to help.

Most children entered the institute between four and seven years old. Many were under four. The main reason for their institutionalisation was that they posed a danger to themselves and others, which was seen as scandalous.

The physicians of the Centro di Igiene Mentale (Mental Health Centre) or of the Clinica Universitaria di Neuropsichiatria infantile (University Clinic of Pediatric Psychiatry) diagnosed them as dangerous. This diagnosis was both a testimony to a repressive ideology and a cynical expression of a *fictio juris* (legal fiction) to have the hospital fees refunded.

The inhumane conditions led the nurses to protect themselves and reduce their affective investments. Some often chose the most beautiful or quietest or most obedient child in the ward, who could be the object of a special affective relationship. They treated her or him as a daughter or a son and tended to her or him exclusively. It was a defence mechanism of scotomisation in response to the problems and contradictions of the ward. This mechanism of isolation led some nurses to become emotionally attached to a single child and exclude all the others (Psichiatria Democratica, 1975).

Work in the children's ward was experienced as so frustrating and unsatisfying that, when personnel had to go to work there, even for a temporary substitution, they considered it a punishment. Sometimes management used it in this manner against the personnel.

Most of the children showed severe psychophysical deficits necessitating integrated rehabilitation programs. Unfortunately, in these conditions, personnel inertly added to a progressive worsening of the deficit. Perversely, the idea that these children could not be cured was reinforced.

At the phantasmatic level, the contact with a child with a severe deficit can provoke intense fears of regressing to primitive phases and a deep identity crisis in the health-care workers, who risk not feeling that their presence and existential borders are confirmed and safe.

The parents of the disabled children reacted to their guilt and suffering due to the difficult acceptance of their child's limits in two extreme manners, delimiting a *continuum* of pathological reaction: strong abnegation and complete and exclusive dedication to their child; or explicit intolerance towards their child and an almost irresistible impulse to deny the parent-child relationship (Solnit and Stark, 1961).

Because it was impossible to gain significative results in everyday work or the worsening of the psychomotor condition of the child, the institution defended itself from the frustration and the deep sense of guilt of its health-care workers in a radical way: by resorting to repression. This defence mechanism leads to the faultless idea that these children cannot recover in any way. Primitive and archaic defence mechanisms dominate the hospital system, so that resistance to change is deep and hard. These defences are very similar to those that can be observed in certain patients functioning with primitive defences, which are generally classified as paranoid-schizoid (Dartington et al., 1992).

The rehabilitation intervention with children having serious deficits would need a kind of relationship patiently promoting personal autonomy at all levels (motor, alimentary, sphincter, social). This autonomy can be approached and sometimes gained only with a constantly active presence, stimulations, and attentions in key moments of the day, with a special attention to meals and the toilet.

The educational intervention the institution chose was to establish a traditional school, whose didactics did not consider the real existential experience of the child, the fundamental relevance of emotions in the affective development, the motivation to learn, or the need of highly individualised relationships, despite the many efforts of the schoolmistresses. The program mocked the traditional didactics and, at best, could lead to dogmatism, superficial factual knowledge, and authoritarianism. Nonetheless, as adults many of these children now recall with pleasure the schoolmistress, the uniform, their desk, and the schoolroom with pleasure. They exhibit the same nostalgia of anyone who remembers and transforms (of course with a certain degree of idealisation) the crucial moments of their childhood, often in contrast with the misery of the present.

In the Nativity Scene, this feeling of nostalgia can be seen in the various representations of the children's ward and the school. The former is crude and graphic: it is a highly realistic image of the institutional atmosphere. The children's poses are representations of autism, but also of abandonment and relational isolation; the play of lights, perspectives, and distances clearly express the gloomy environmental squalor. Although the nun is at the centre of the scene, she is not only spatially but also emotionally far from the children who are dressed in pink and white checkered shirts. The children are left alone in a too wide, cold, and bare environment to promote any affective relationships (Figure 9.1).

The representation of the classroom exhibits the warmth of the nostalgic transfiguration. The spectators, above all the old ones, can easily recognise themselves with their aprons and the bow around their necks, sitting at the desk, listening to the schoolmistress who speaks between the desk and blackboard. The classroom of the asylum school could look like that of any primary school 50 years ago (Figure 9.2).

However, this special school did not stimulate children with intuitive, concrete, expressive, creative, or dynamic activities leading to an increasing degree of symbolisation, that is, activities promoting a sense of freedom, relativity, and existential maturation. The lack of involvement of the ward's personnel maintained a guardianship attitude that reinforced the split between the inside and outside and the idea that the school experience was useless, unable to improve living conditions. The fact that the school offered to the children few existential opportunities that inevitably disappeared after the doors of the ward closed behind

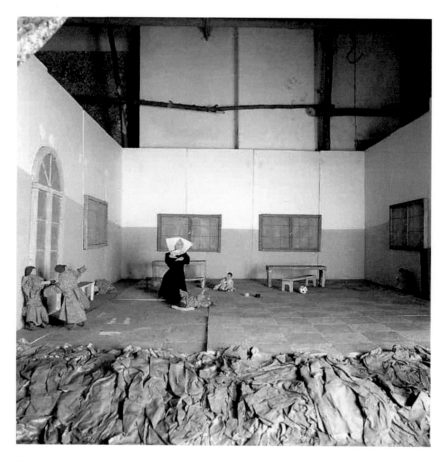

Figure 9.1 The children's ward.

them was a source of frustration and disappointment, sometimes causing reactive and particularly aggressive behaviours.

At the end of their study on the psychiatric hospital, Stanton and Schwartz (1954) point out that the traditional institutional treatment tends to result in forms of apathy and affective retreat in the adult and minor patients, who become bored with and disinvested in the personnel.

In his "Relazione del Bilancio Annuale" (report of the annual balance) (1925) the director of the asylum of Cogoleto describes the children's ward in total contrast to the most basic norms of objectivity and intellectual honesty. In fact, he writes that Ward No. 10 is a small and elegant space with verandas for the little halfwits. According to him, the ward is a point of pride for the administration because it is one of the few in Italy that provides these disgraced children (separated from the adults) with an appropriate, comfortable, and happy environment. Here the minds of

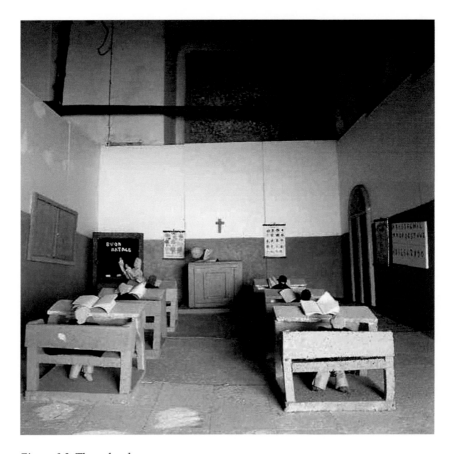

Figure 9.2 The school.

these children, which an unkind nature had denied joys and reasons to live by dulling their senses or delaying or even preventing their perceptions, can receive an adequate education and instruction. Here everything works to repair the injustice of this nature: inside and outside the ward, everything is a smile, a joy of colours, organisation, and cleanliness. Two kind nuns compensate for the maternal deficiencies and use funds from their simple and excellent charity to help the children. The nurses, almost all war widows, transform themselves into tender mothers for these derelict children.

Today the children of the past, now adults in various wards, present a worsening of their original psychomotor deficits and personality traits typical of those who have been forced into a very precocious institutionalisation. These traits can be summarised in this way (Petrella, 1993f):

• superficial social contacts

- disaffection, hypo-affection, lability of emotional ties, tendency to isolation, aggressiveness, a-sociality
- a tendency to pretend, to lie (even in improbable and fantastic manners), to steal (Bowlby, 1951)
- frustrating impossibility to those trying to help them, incapacity to accept any affect
- personal identity disorder (Bender, 1947)
- deficiency of temporalisation.

Their disorganised adaptation makes the patients victims of contrasting sensations of desire and fear, so that they adopt a discontinuous attitude made of approaches and departures.

The patients make iterative requests to the psychiatric hospital, which becomes the place of their acting-out. They consider the same person good today and bad tomorrow and basically do not trust anyone: no one is relevant in their lives. The traumatic experiences due to violence or carelessness interiorise the violent and disturbed objects that, at the same time, become the receptacle of the projective destructivity of the individual (Steiner, 1993).

The incapacity to accept the affects can be due to the threat against the very frail positive maternal object, which can be maintained at the price of projecting outside the aggression originally directed against it.

The responses of the health-care workers swing between a repairing anxiety and a deep frustration, especially when the attempts at contact increase. The consequence is an authoritarian solution that leads to protests and sensational actions such as attempts to escape or self-harm that, at last, provoke novel segregations and containments. In these situations, patients attempt to actively provoke that frustration that they are afraid to passively suffer, as Freud (1920b) described in children's play.

The complexity of these institutional dynamics stresses the need for a continuative and specific personal training and teamwork that allows the expression and working through of emotional and relational difficulties.

In the last years various projects of institutional reanimation and integrated rehabilitation started. They establish both the fundamental physiotherapy support for the disabled and attention to the creative skills of patients via pottery and literacy courses for adults. The main aim is to learn from past mistakes and thus truly allow the development of autonomy, by maintaining a constant collaboration between teachers and staff. Even experiences of motor education and resocialisation (also through play) started: they aim to prevent the institution from failing again and exercise the developmental skills of the patients. The latter is to give patients the possible chance of being socially accepted outside the institution. This is a difficult task because health-care workers must avoid, however, raising false hopes, which if dashed, would cause the small glimmers laboriously opened to close again immediately (Barisone and Schinaia, 1995).

Rehabilitation projects must not try to repair a flaw or fill a void, rather they ought to reinsert the patients in a circle of interests and desires that were impeded by the destruction that characterised their development and made it highly disharmonic (Petrella, 1993b).

10 Work

In Christian-Medieval culture, richness and poverty were not linked to work-related activities, and thus they were not seen as social phenomena. Instead, they were considered complementary elements of a providential design. The rich and poor were reciprocally necessary: charity, more specifically almsgiving, elevated the poor from their material misery and simultaneously enabled the rich to redeem themselves from their mortal sins by engaging in merciful behaviour (Duby, 1973).

When famine and other unfavourable conditions began to affect many segments of a population, the problems of begging and pauperism assumed scary social dimensions that caused a crisis in the Christian ethics of poverty. The figure of the poor began to lose every link with the sacred and instead started to be seen as a threat to the social order.

The insufficiency of philanthropy and private charity caused the creation of various secular and ecclesial institutions (hospitals, hospices, charities) for the poor, always swinging between the polarities of assistance and repression (Gutton, 1974).

Poverty as a social condition was no longer exalted. Instead it was stigmatised as voluntary elusion from the work commitments. Assistance and relief, once a right of the poor, became a duty and an obligation to safeguard the security of the state. Thus, those who did not meet this obligation were repressed (Geremek, 1973).

It was not until the end of the Middle Ages and the beginning of the Modern Age that misery began to be considered a social phenomenon. There was a shift from Christian philanthropy to the economic politics of the Industrial Age. It tried to solve the problem of misery with work and occupation, by emanating social laws and inventing practises such as ergotherapy and proposing ways of resocialization based on the work (Romano C., 1990).

Work in the asylums seemed to be an efficacious tool of social control and a disciplinary practise perfect for the pre-industrial state's economy. But what was confounded with the state's assistance was neither work performance nor a product but the statement of a value, the acceptance of work as an ethical prescription (Geremek, 1986). With the birth of the

DOI: 10.4324/9781003381723-10

asylums, work fully acquired a disciplinary function and became part of an ergotherapeutic project.

Inside the reclusive institutions the obligation to work had a rehabilitative function, in some moments as a form of redemption, in others as a form of therapy. But behind the different ideological justifications, there was always a need for social control in generalising the obligation to work and imposing it as a basic disciplinary principle (Romano C., 1992).

People were put away in psychiatric hospitals not to be cured but to be disciplined: the evidence is the high number of hospitalisations lasting far longer than the required cure. No therapeutic project but only a pedagogy oriented to moral treatment could justify this exceeding time of hospitalisation (Romano C., 1994).

The early 19th century brought the completion of a process which began in the Renaissance and continued through the Calvinist ethics and the Industrial Revolution: to gradually attribute to work an absolute social value (Accornero, 1980). That was the beginning of the first studies and theories about the usefulness of work in curing the mentally ill. (Pinel, 1801) argued that work is a fundamental law in the treatment of in-patients. In 1813, Tuke argued that perhaps one of the most efficacious tools to stimulate self-control in patients is regular work. Work in the fields is always beneficial and promotes recovery and healing. In 1830, Todd strongly recommended to the family of a patient discharged from the Hartford Retreat in Connecticut (US) the benefits of, as well as the need for, regular work as something offering the expectation of a modest but fair reward for being hardworking and judicious.

In the 1920s the German psychiatrist Simon, a supporter of eugenic and racist ideas and Nazism, promoted ergotherapy as a discipline. It was considered a method of "more active therapy" (*Aktivere Krankenbehandlung*) able to improve the physical (increase in sleep, appetite, strength, and muscle flexibility) and psychological conditions (decrease in mental damage and aggression) of patients who were considered no longer as sick but productive, and from whom the administration could gain a certain economic advantage (Walter, 2002).

Psychiatrists after Simon accepted his ergotherapeutic ideology and divided patients in three main classes: those who could be cured via other means to "reintegrate" in society as soon as possible; those who had to be locked up as passive objects of assistance; and those who would slowly acquire their freedom inside the hospital by working in and for the institution, thus reintegrating and adapting themselves to the institutional micro-society (Benevelli, 1996).

The term "ergotherapy" (from the Ancient Greek *ergon*, meaning "work" or "opus") became associated to the so-called occupational therapy in the asylums. In general, the term "ergotherapy" indicated all the cures through the means of work responding to the patient's need to be outside the closed wards for a few hours a day, no matter for which activity, whereas occupational therapy proper was not a ritual and immutable practise, but tended to consider the instable needs of the patient and, aiming at placing the patient in the working context, it considered work as a sort of entity having an intrinsic therapeutic power (Cerati, 1993). It aimed to stimulate individual creativity but was limited to the context of the asylum. It was not open to social and professional reintegration (Jolivet, 1981).

The beginning of ergotherapeutic proposals coincided with what happened in prisons, when it was decided that punishment had to include the possibility of economic and social redemption. This promoted senseless and aimless work like the grotesque parody of the work exalted in the slogan on the entrance of Auschwitz, "Arbeit macht frei" ("work sets you free").

One of the aims of ergotherapy was to tyre the patients. According to the pedagogical assumptions of the time, if they were tired they could make less use of their sexuality. Later ergotherapy was considered a re-educational method of the mind to give to the patient his sociability, that is, his readjustment to the outside collective life and to counter his tendency to retreat and isolate himself due to inactivity or morbid fantasies (De Giacomo, 1960).

Following the psychopathology related to the passions, the distraction of thought from imaginative activity was not considered the outcome or the start of a slow way back to re-establish communication with the others; rather, it was assumed to be the source of psychopathology, literally following the Bible's proverb "Idle hands are the devil's workshop," as if idleness could make one fantasise and thus drive him mad (Peloso, 1992).

As a first-person instrument of cure as well as a guardian, the nurse had to understand that the work was useful also for those who produced very little because of idleness but that, when they were taken from this condition and the consequent dehumanisation, they received the same benefits of their active companions.

Later ergotherapy was intended as a means of resocialization and re-learning of the correct social manners, a transitive communication activity, a medium of interpersonal relationships, a possibility to improve perception and self-acceptance in a wider human dimension, a discharge and channelling of aggression towards inanimate objects and not towards subjects, a concrete approach to reality by manipulating objects, an offer to experience her or his possibility and promote a better definition of personality by stimulation self-management and autonomy (Pedrinoni and Tarantola, 1971). There were many ways to put ergotherapy in practise (Romano C., 1994):

1 assigning the patient to increasingly difficult work
2 according to the patient's psychomotor skills, choosing stimulating or sedative (monotonous and stereotyped) work

3 trying to re-educate the patient to his original profession
4 especially for young patients, trying to teach new work.

If mental disease is disorder and irregularity, nothing is better than routine, monotonous, and regular work to restore the lost or never possessed order or define a new one. Work is considered a form of discipline that the patient must internalise so much that he will feel it as a need.

The organisation of ergotherapy was very strict. It followed these modalities:

1 Internal or indoor ergotherapy, occurring inside specific rooms in the wards. The recommended jobs for men were weaving wicker and raffia, cardboard setting up brooms and brushes, artisanal painting, sculpture, modelling—all the jobs that do not require complicated or demanding equipment. In the same manner, the recommended jobs for women were sewing, mending, embroidery, knitting, and making curtains and carpets
2 Workshop ergotherapy. These were workshops strictly linked to the hospital's general services, carpentry, shoemaking, printing, bookbinding, pottery, weaving, laundry, ironing, tailoring, blacksmithing, and mechanical work
3 External or outdoor ergotherapy. This included agricultural, horticultural, gardening, and preparation of sports fields. It was useful for the progress of agriculture and the evolution of agricultural techniques. When agricultural work was instituted in the asylums, there was significant improvement in the breeding of poultry and other animals, the construction of pigsties, the production of milk, etc.

There are different scenes in the Nativity Scene of Cogoleto dedicated to work. This indicates how much the institution invested in ergotherapy, especially in the workshops and outdoor ergotherapy, and how important work was in the collective imagery of the psychiatric population. This was valid both for the patients and nurses, all of whom had peasant and artisan origins and thus were sympathetic to the type of work that was done at the institution.

The scenes of the Nativity Scene are also an important historical document about the kinds of work techniques that were typical at the beginning of the previous century. These conserved techniques bring to mind dialects in immigrant communities in foreign countries. Both have been substituted by newer techniques or linguistic expressions, but in the contexts of the psychiatric hospital and immigrant communities they still exist.

The scenes of the kitchen, carpentry workshop, and laundry (Figures 10.1–10.3) significantly express the full-time use of patients as a critical cog in the complex institutional machine. Hygienic conditions and injury prevention are not considered at all.

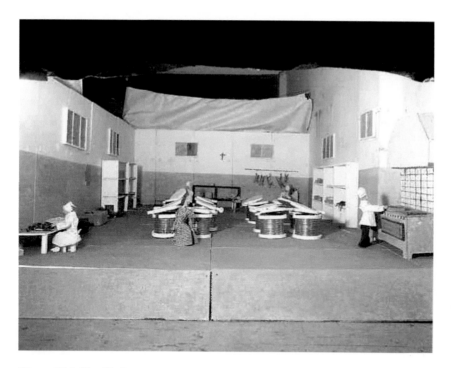

Figure 10.1 The kitchens.

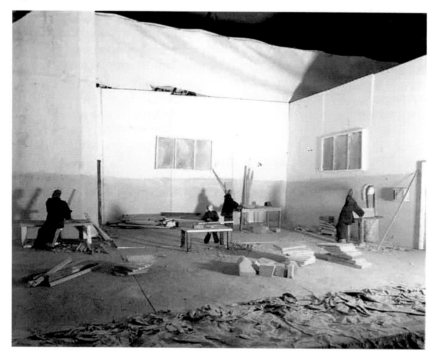

Figure 10.2 The carpentry workshop.

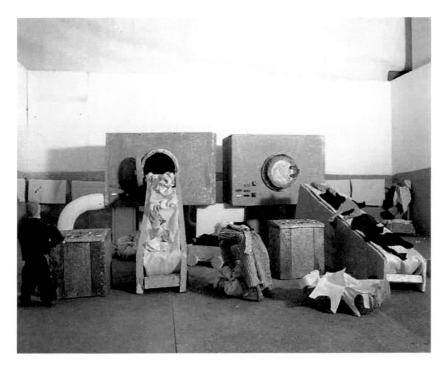

Figure 10.3 The laundry.

Thanks to ergotherapy, the psychiatric institution's economics improved significantly, to the point where it became almost self-sufficient, and the work function of the patients became almost irreplaceable, mainly thanks to the low management costs and remarkable profit. For example, the typography of the asylum of Cogoleto (Figure 10.4), which was located exactly where the Nativity Scene was built, supplied the administration with all its forms and publications, including the scientific journal of the hospital. It also printed a small journal for the patients, strongly characterised by moralistic and paternalistic tones.

The scene of the pigsty is part of the wider rural context, composed of cultivated terraces, olive trees, and fruit trees (Figures 10.5–10.10). It represents the utopia of outdoor agricultural work that redeems the patients from the unworthy status of fools and elevates them (of course, by continuing to maintain a neat separation from the external world) to the condition of workers, a condition considered *per se* to be the ethical but not the economic symbol of deliverance from evil.

According to Simon (Walter, 2002), through ergotherapy, the sick person should have gained his freedom, working without a contract to later be able to stipulate a real work contract, but only when released, at some unspecified future time.

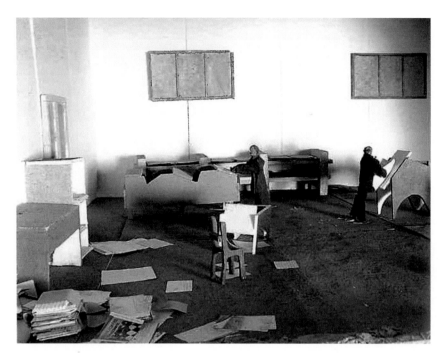

Figure 10.4 The typography.

Where once patients were paid in kind (with cigarettes, wine, sweets), they now received paper money valid only within the hospital, or credits in an account at the treasurer's office. From his account, the patient could periodically withdraw small sums and possibly leave a larger part to be collected after his discharge.

Hochmann (1971) argues that the salary was introduced to justify the importance of the work in the asylums because therapeutic motivation alone was not sufficient. But this salary is fake; it is grotesque. The salary in the hospital is a remuneration having nothing to do with the social dimensions of a real salary. Money trafficking inside a totalitarian institution is just a game, like the board game Monopoly, a simulacrum of the exchanges outside every social circuit of production, distribution, and consumption. Only this circuit can establish a commercial value. The exchange occurs in a context of the exclusion of the value. What is exchanged is a thing against another thing that does not represent anything if not the grotesque materialisation of the exchange gesture.

On the one hand, the work activity of the patient can be a spontaneous social action and, for this reason, mainly therapeutic; on the other hand, it is always a real working force, energy produced that cannot be alienated only through a free contract or by imposition. About this contradiction,

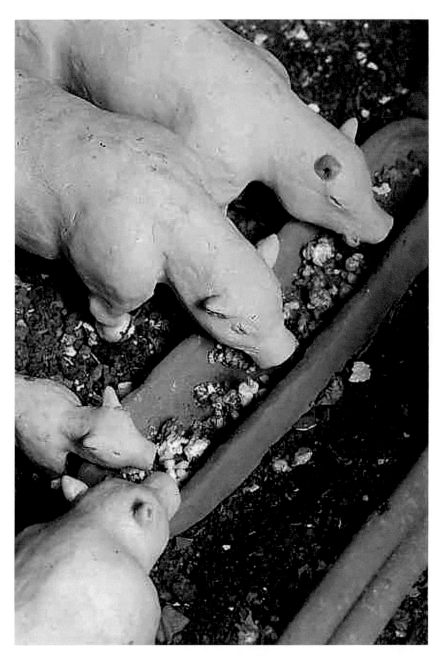

Figure 10.5 The pigsty (detail).

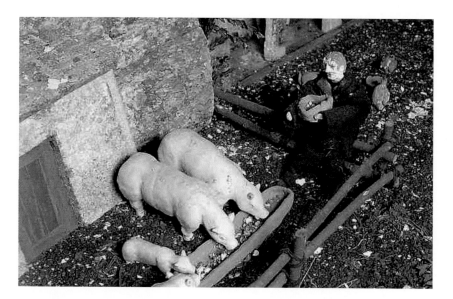

Figure 10.6 The pigsty (detail).

the institution has always been ambiguous because it has always needed the two main features of work: its therapeutic aspect to move the patient's active participation in the therapeutic interaction, and its workforce aspect able to move and keep alive the functioning of the institutional mechanism (Slavich and Jervis Comba, 1973).

In a critical assessment of the ergotherapeutic practise, it would be unfair to not recognise its historical merit to have humanised at least some areas of the asylum and mitigated the violence of the patients' segregation at least in certain circumstances. This could have been done through the strong link between ergotherapy and the transformation of the asylum according to the principles of "moral treatment," the *no restraint*, something not always put into practise. Certainly, there was labour exploitation. But it is not enough to explain all the phenomena: the idea that internment and ergotherapy had to be the components of a massive project based on a low-cost workforce is naïve and false. In fact, when the asylum did not suffer economic losses, its unpaid labour force of patients guaranteed the institution's financial self-sufficiency (Peloso, 1992).

Some features of the work such as fatigue, constraint, and normative conformism can give an order to the instinctual world of the psychotic through the mechanism of repression or, above all, the split of emotional parts that cannot be easily integrated. This appears to have worked in the asylum's ergotherapeutic practise by promoting that residual evolution or social healing that is the declared target of many treatments. In this sense, the psychotic can benefit (perhaps only superficially) from the work

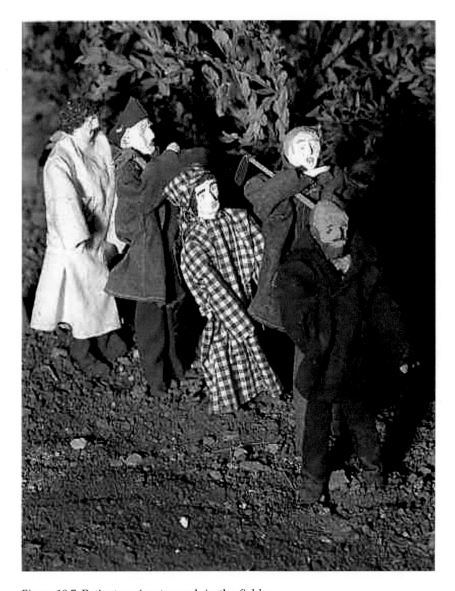

Figure 10.7 Patients going to work in the fields.

practise if he uses it as a defence against himself. It is a sort of social straitjacket connecting his split parts (it is unknown for how long) (Cerati, 1993).

In Italy, the writings of Basaglia and his followers sharply criticised ergotherapeutic ideology and gave a new outlook to the patients' working activities by creating work cooperatives. These criticisms put

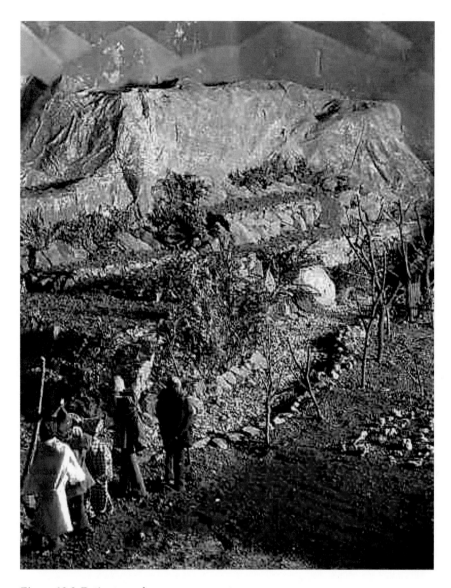

Figure 10.8 Patients as farmers.

into question the entire institution and as a consequence the ergotherapeutic ideology of work, as something collusive, often solitary, denying
the internal world and considering the emotions of the other as a danger
to be avoided, authoritatively demanding homologation and obedience,
always the same throughout the years, without a perspective of professional or relational development, necessary only to distract from the

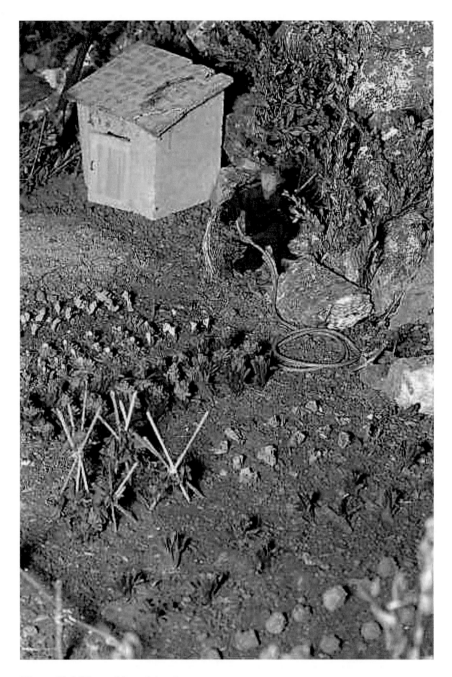

Figure 10.9 Vegetable cultivation.

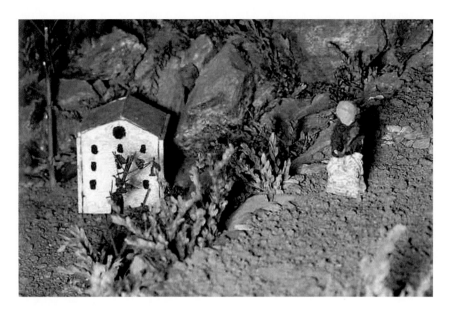

Figure 10.10 Woman sitting in a field.

universe of the patients' internal worlds through fatigue (Peloso, 1992). The creation of the cooperative was a challenge because it symbolised a meeting point between apparent opposites: production and inability, free market and assistance, business and solidarity, work and participation, social integration and ghettoization, public and private. In the cooperatives the power of solidarity acts as a transformative power along with money and technical and administrative power. It fosters rights and responsibilities influencing the life quality of a community (Righetti and Rotelli, 1990).

Working entails selling goods belonging to us, realising a responsibility for submission, a professionality for the institutional incapacity, relationships for solitude.

The strategies of social entrepreneurship are different, even the opposite, of ergotherapy. Even if it were an issue of moral treatment of the deviances, in that case the method is not to make the patients work, but put them in the best economical, organisational, and relational conditions to do it. This is because the "treatment" does not aim to normalise, but to rebuild people's confidence and self-respect, integrity, and complexity: freedom, autonomy, and responsibility develop through their use and practise (De Leonardis et al., 1994). Social entrepreneurship represents an experiment trying to develop a web of material and symbolic exchanges between cure and free market, approaching and transforming some features of both these systems (De Leonardis and Emmenegger, 2005).

According to Freud (1930, p. 80), *no other technique for the conduct of life attaches the individual so firmly to reality as laying emphasis on work; for his work at least gives him a secure place in a portion of reality, in the human community.*

The term "cooperative" literally means a collective kind of entrepreneurship, different from other types of entrepreneurship because of its mutualistic and non-lucrative ends of the "partners." This juridical definition does not contradict the political-anthropological reference to a model of economic development contrasting the dehumanisation of the profit logic. According to this perspective, the therapeutic function consists of a new form of contract, that permits interpersonal relationships that were difficult, impossible, or meaningless before (Balduzzi, 1989).

Warner (1985) posits that, according to results of clinical studies, psychotic patients who work tend to avoid a new hospitalisation longer than unemployed ones do. These results make one think (but do not demonstrate) that work is the cause for the patients' improvement.

Empirical evidence shows that unemployment has enduring and clear psychopathological effects on a patient, such as depression, anxiety, and generalised stress leading to a strong reduction of self-esteem (Crepet, 1990).

It is possible to organise worker cooperatives with the most seriously ill patients as long as the work requires no sacrifices or a constant effort in rigidly set tasks.

If the long years of isolation and inactivity tend to determine a total loss of the patient's identity, it is necessary to stimulate the most basic and fundamental mechanisms for the stability of the Ego, stimulating the exercise of its functions and strengthening the sense of identity. They need time, the time to observe the new situation to assess if it is trustworthy and not dangerous for their mental and physical stability. They need exceptional work, freely chosen and free to be left and taken again, leaving room to fantasy, almost play, something becoming creative and able to slowly connect who practises it and the external work, without categorical commitments (Izzo, 1983). Work activities for hospitalised patients must occur outside the institution, beyond the walls of the psychiatric hospital. There are occupational activities that occur and must occur inside the institution, the psychiatric hospital, and the mental health centre. However, they are something completely different from true working activities: they are the first steps of a rehabilitation process, those in which the problem is faced and tested and the basis for the future is defined (Colafelice, 1993).

In *Civilization and Its Discontents* (1930, p. 80), Freud writes: *Professional activity is a source of special satisfaction if it is freely chosen, if ... it makes possible the use of existing inclinations or persisting or constitutionally reinforced instinctual impulses.*

In *The Monkey's Wrench* (1978), Primo Levi argues that we can and must fight so that the outcome of work remains in the hands of those who perform it, and that work itself is not a punishment. But love, or conversely hatred, for work is an inner and original fact, strongly depending upon the history of the individual and less than is believed upon the productive structures in which work occurs.

The main activity with the most seriously deconstructed patients is the imitation of emotionally significant figures (for example, the nurses), who represent a constant and safe point of reference. But this imitation must not be considered the final and desired effect of learning, but rather a necessary and intermediate phase in the constitutive process of the identity (Tagliabue, 1993).

According to Gaddini (1984), the most common error is to believe that the mental operation of imitation involves nothing but repeating what another person does to reach a certain aim. In humankind, this occurs only when imitation is integrated with the push to internalise, that is, with introjection. It is the integration of imitation and introjection that leads to the most evolved capacity of identification.

There are two main kinds of job placement:

- socialising placement allows patient to communicate with reality thanks to the strong mediation of the health-care workers. The activities are simple, manual, or recreational. The degree of protection of the work experience is very high so as not to grant excessive autonomy to the patient. In fact, too much autonomy can result in a massive regression when the patient anxiously feels that they are failing
- true job placement requires the emotional presence of the health-care workers but is for those patients who exhibit a higher degree, autonomy, and dexterity.

The move from the first to the second kind of job placement can be seen as a passage of a developmental phase of the same patient's existence. The socialisation phase is introductory and creates the conditions for a true working phase (Schinaia et al., 1985; Schinaia, 2023b).

The clinical picture and thus the prognosis are assumed to be as very vague and not rigid assessment criteria. This is because it was demonstrated that some severely schizophrenic patients can slowly but progressively improve and reach acceptable degrees of autonomy and self-realisation.

At least two cases must be distinguished for those suffering from severe mental diseases:

- those who have never been paid for work for various reasons, for example a highly disabling mental disease since they were children or adolescents. This is the case of people highly dependent on their families or assistance structures, often having had early and prolonged experiences of hospitalisation and an early diagnosis defining their invalidity (and often any form of carer's allowance), showing low levels of education and very poor autonomous social relationships. These are not "falls" or "failures" because school, social, and work contexts are not strongly integrated. Because of this condition, none, not even the patient himself, asks or expects to be paid.

- those who have been paid for work but who lost it for various reasons, for example, the onset of a mental disease hindering work commitments. These are "falls" or "failures" not only in the social and work integration but also in the attempts, challenges, and experiences. The person knows how to perform and maintain paid work (Benevelli, 1996).

Liberman (1988) distinguishes between nonspecific group activities, which aim to invite the patients to socialise, and activities using techniques for learning specific behaviours in a systematic manner. These techniques require a therapeutic alliance with the patient and his family and the definition of shared goals to reach.

The cooperative's product-work carried and valued in society and the rediscovery of at least partial working capacities of the patients are the concrete, achievable, and clearly assessable goals compensating also that frustration that the chronic disease causes in the health-care workers. This frustration is a consequence of the fact that the product-health in its entirety cannot be reached (Izzo and Lucchi, 1991).

Jaques (1970) argues that work is an exercise of discretion within the prescribed limitations to reach an object. It is something assessable through a reality check and by maintaining at the same time the working through of the consequent anxiety.

The growth of Ego strength comes from the ability to experience uncertainties, lost opportunities, or errors. It is at the basis of that constructive self-criticism that leads one to learn from one's errors.

Fornari (1976) stresses the growth function of the work experience and its organisation. This function mediates between reality and the primary persecutory anxieties. It implies solitude and uncertainty about the outcome of a certain project and thus can promote the achievement of more mature positions. Working is the passage from the "wood" of pregenitality to the "field" of genitality, in which the wood represents all the irrational unconscious processes (the private symbol) and the field all the rational conscious processes (the object produced or accepted by others) (Stella, 1983).

The meaning and proposal of work for schizophrenics can be also seen as the attempt to restore a transition experience. In fact, the work of schizophrenics does not take place in a shared reality: it is like the play, and thus occurs in the transitional space, whose non-constitution causes an irreparable rupture of that feeling of continuity of the existence at the basis of mental health (Winnicott, 1951).

Thus, the work can be a way to reach the external reality that was inaccessible to the schizophrenic patient because of his mechanisms of split, narcissistic withdrawal, and denial. It is important that the health-care workers can change their internal image of the schizophrenic patients to make this reality accessible (Izzo and Lucchi, 1991).

Meltzer (1973) points out that in the childish organisation of the Self, the Ego is in a primary relationship with the Id and this results in play, whereas, vice versa, in the adult organisation, the adult part of the Ego is in a mediate relationship with the Id through projective identification and this results in work. Here Meltzer reconsiders one of the themes of Ego Psychology, that about the evolution from play to work, from a different perspective.

Play and work are specific and temporarily different moments of psychological development. A too neat distinction between them can lead to splits at the individual level. These splits are incompatible with the creation of a healthy personal identity. At the general level, this means that an excessive distinction between work and play can confirm that lack of flexibility in work and that experiences of discomfort that persons and social observers often complain about (Stella, 1983).

It is true that in therapeutic work with psychotics it is important to do things together. But it is also true that these things must remain activities having a strong symbolic value. Their function is to help patient to reactivate a creative process and not to fill a void that must be filled or repair a damage that must be repaired (Hochmann, 1982).

For the psychotic patient, the "good enough" therapist must accept the temporary condition of "working appearance." This acceptance has a twofold function: first, it preserves that omnipotent nucleus that the limitations of every effective work or activity can attack by challenging the magnificent image of the patient; second, it promotes the potential for the patient's emancipation, based on a safety coming from the acceptance of his deficit and, at the same time, on the recognition of the need of an illusory area functioning as a "prosthesis" of the deficit itself (Bordi et al., 1995).

Staff's giving has a dual statute: first, as it often happens, it represents the chance of indefinitely continuing a total proxy and dependence from the others; second, in a completely different interpretation, it represents the need to communicate to the patient the reassuring presence of Another open to give so that he can rediscover the capacity to take (Ferro et al., 1995).

Moving from activity to activism or permitting that a form of manic behaviour takes the place of enthusiasm are dangerous defensive attitudes to protect from the panic emerging from the feeling of being invaded or drained or, on the contrary, useless and impotent, something typical when meeting with a psychotic person.

Patience and graduality are the basic conditions so that the temporary states of mourning (Jaques, 1970), connected to sensations of inability, limitation, and tendency to err, can be slowly experienced and then tolerated, without reaching a pseudo-normality consisting of busyness without reflection. This pseudo-normality can lead the patient to catastrophic falls difficult to work through or to definitively leave the work experience because it is assumed to be excessively frustrating.

According to Correale (1991), a pure and too restrictive rehabilitative model tends to follow a pedagogic-behaviouristic logic. Within this logic, the patient is a person who is receiving those possibilities (especially in socialisation) that he did not have in life and who must be taught to perform professional, artisanal, or artistic functions that had been lost in the process that made the disease chronic. An approach of this kind does not consider two fundamental points: first, insisting only on the healthy side of the patient, which is something valid *per se*, can increase the splitting mechanisms, so that the patient can create a false self, adapting to the demands of the context, but that it is separated from his dramatic and suffering internal nucleus; second, because the drama of this kind of patient is his weakness in the cohesive force of the self, every therapy must consider this fundamental aspect more than practical and behavioural performances.

The desire to work cannot be presupposed: it must be construed and found together, otherwise the different rehabilitative programs focused on the work are doomed to failure. The techniques used in these programs must be integrated with the creative features of the curing art.

In a process of helping to individuate and strengthen the working capacities of people with severe psychiatric diseases it is not important to recognise that "the work is a therapy" (something present also in ergotherapy; rather, it is fundamental to individuate and practise those therapeutic and social interventions fostering the insertion or the reinsertion of these people in the world of work, a world of exchanges and relationships (Spinelli, 1995).

Thus, rehabilitation must be considered as a specific moment of activation or as the final moment inside a unique therapeutic process mainly based on the interpersonal and developmental relationship.

11   Death

In so-called archaic societies, every aspect of the ritual system referred to a collective representation of death, and all knowledge about it was based on ritualisation. On the contrary, today there is often a dissociation between the ritualised aspect of death and its collective representation. Such a representation is now secularised and largely explainable in medical terms (Papi, 1980).

The archaic human being was a stakeholder of his own death. Dying was not the moment of death *per se*: it was a part of a process, a socially established passage that did not deny life but brought about a new life, another and different one (Fuchs, 1969).

The main defence mechanisms from death and the dead were obsessivity, displacement, the illusion of rendering something eternal, and ingesting the corpse.

For the Medieval human being, death was tame, not wild. Sudden and violent death was considered a shame and a disgrace (Ariès, 1974).

In the Renaissance, death was not simply conceived as a conclusion from being but a separation from owning material goods or even having a personal history. Some essays on the art of dying began to be published, and biographies became popular. Death went from being conceived as sleep or rest to a physical degradation, suffering, and decomposition.

In the 17th century, death was no longer considered shameful. People hoped for a sudden death. In the 17th and 18th centuries, the physician first supported and then substituted for the clergy of the Middle Ages and Renaissance as a witness of the final event.

The 17th century physician considered the time of death as a state belonging to both life and death, and death as something definitive only in the moment of decomposition. By the 19th century, death did not last more time than a geometric point acquires density and thickness: it was nothing but a broken-down machine (Ariès, 1977).

The 19th century saw novels full of descriptions of beautiful deaths: they were a clear falsehood given the anxiety behind the ineffability and inexpressibility of it. Until the first years of the 20th century, death was a social and public event, especially in small urban areas.

DOI: 10.4324/9781003381723-11

The participation of relatives and acquaintances was intense and stressed the sense of community, the belonging and sharing of the dying person's pain, and the mourning of his family. Every death touched every one and, as Flaubert used to say, added a tomb in that necropolis that is the human heart (Steegmuller, 1980).

The funeral reception luncheon had both the sense of cannibalistic re-incorporation of the still-warm corpse, a ritual heritage of archaic societies, and the sense of taking care of the relatives who were broken and weakened from the pain and, in the first phase of mourning, thereby unable to satisfy even basic needs such as eating.

In cities today there is no sign of what happened. Where once upon a time the old hearse passed, with the slow and sad procession of relatives and friends behind it, the shop doors shut out of respect for the deceased and the mourning, today the hearse is nothing but an ordinary black car which anonymously gets lost in the flow of traffic at dawn, before people go to work.

Contemporary society does not take a rest or pause. The death of an individual does not touch its continuity. In the cities, all goes on as if no one really dies. Unsaid and unspoken, death is pushed into a clandestine state. The sick does not want to know about it and the relatives, the physician, the priest must not say anything about it. The dying and those surrounding them play along with the comedy of "nothing changed," "life continues as before," and "all is still possible." The time of the last goodbyes no longer exists. Once many people visited the room of the dying; now the mere idea of entering a room that reeks of sweat and urine is intolerable. Above all, children must be kept away from death. This is a new image of death: the ugly and hidden death, hidden because it is ugly and dirty (Ariès, 1977).

Galimberti (1997) argues that the issue about death is not regretting the lack of collective rituals but rather that understanding why these rites are no longer necessary because for us, today, death changed in thickness and density. Now our survival depends much more on our work, our skills, and our relationships with the living rather than on the recurrence of the memory of the dead.

Although it is necessary that nostalgic thoughts led and forced us improperly, it must be recognised that the hospital had been the institutional place in which the experience of death has been seized. Here death became a mere clinical fact, a simple impossibility of life because it was masked; it was no longer public—it was solitary.

Mourning disappears: people refuse to participate in death for fear of naming it. In *Mourning and Melancholia*, Freud (1917) distinguishes between those two. The former is the intrapsychic process of coping with the loss of a loved one. During this process, the subject divests of the external world for a time and falls back on his inner resources. This reaction is characterised by that sadness experienced during a separation.

Divestment of the lost object by withdrawing libido is part of the mourning process. A process of displacement frees the subject from the clutches of the object.

The work of mourning occurs through a progressive and painful detachment from the emotional investments of the lost object. It is an internal working through of the contradictory aspects (libidinal, but also aggressive) that these investments reveal. In the more mature forms of working through, the work of mourning involves acquiring the skill to find in the internal dimension of the relationship with what had been lost in the external one. Tolerating separation, loss of objects, or, very briefly, death itself, is a skill. The ability to love is the most authentic skill of all. Psychoanalysis allows us to be tragically aware of the ineliminable thickness of the negative, the destruction, the absence, and the pain upon which the possibility to enjoy and love stands out (Barale, 1982).

Freud (1915, p. 299) writes that *no depreciation of feelings of love is intended. (…) Nature (…) contrives to keep love ever vigilant and fresh, so as to guard it against the hate which lurks behind it.*

Today pain and punishment can only be secretly expressed: they must be a private and hidden practice comparable to masturbation (Gorer, 1956). In contemporary societies, death is a taboo like sex was been in the past: it produces similar attitudes of emotional deactivation, concealment, consumerist neutralisation, or pornographic complacency.

Various statistics show that today most people die where they were born, that is, in a hospital. The fact that physicians deal with the concealment of death is only the technological extension of that abandonment that began outside the hospital, that is, in families. Death strongly challenges technical isolation and the system of partial investments typical of the hospital practice. Dying in a hospital ward amplifies deep anxieties and therefore provokes different avoidance and distancing behaviours, sometimes justified by the need to protect the other patients from "distressing" situations and guarantee quiet and peace to the dying. In this manner, the dying person is isolated in a secluded room or sometimes behind a room divider. They are visited as little as possible. The physicians and nurses' interventions become even more technical and subdivided. Because "there is nothing to do," medical examinations decrease in number and take place in an atmosphere of great embarrassment. A "technical" activism substitutes for the relational block around the dying patient. A typical slogan of this activism is "let's keep doing something!"—prescribing drugs that the physicians themselves consider useless and whose aim is to ease the feelings of anxiety, impotence, and guilt of those who witness the death (Barale, 1982).

When we deal with death, we refer to experiences of guilt, cognitive and emotional defeat, and narcissistic wounds to explain some of the attitudes the physicians assume in front of the dying patient. It would be crucial to stress when training medical and paramedical staff that the main aim is not to heal (a phantasm related to the Ego ideal) but to cure (an objectual relation) or to be in a relationship (Berger, 1978).

Just as the most regressed psychotic has a relatively integer part with which we can form an alliance, so, too, the dying person is not just an unsustainable tangle of death anxieties. The dying person has inside himself a part emotionally investing towards the objects and the people of the living world: to interrupt or distort communication with him is to renounce sustaining this part and to help to deal with the fear and anxiety characterising it (Barale, 1982).

As a paradox, next to the clandestine and concealed death in the hospital, an exhibited and spectacularised death can be found: death on television. This can be defined as an epic of the macabre between repression and spectacularisation (Natoli, 1995). This is not only the pompous funeral of important heads of state but also the daily violent death caused by wars, assassinations, massacres, and famines. Televising death on the evening news exhibits the definitive detachment, the total split between the spectacularised event, emphasised without respect or emotional implications. The affective involvement of the spectator becomes distracted and detached, even a form of annoyed co-existence with an event that it is not felt as near but very far, strange, and thus innocuous.

The other side of the coin is that perversion of paying close attention to death: it is the passage from inattention to necrophilia, from lack of *pathos* to excited and voyeuristic observation. Death loses its sacred and terrible character: it is simply ruthless.

In our culture a pseudo-symbolic diction of death is widespread. It denies death and simultaneously desperately looks for the most intellectualised or pornographic versions of death. The epic of the macabre is between pathos and cynicism. Everything is homologated in an irrelevant narrative circularity in which everything has the same value and is indifferent (Corradi Fiumara, 1980).

Death in a psychiatric hospital is an extreme representation of the binomial between the clandestine state and the exhibition typical of present society. The psychiatric hospital assumed a wider historical function than the general hospital: it was the container of the concealment of deviants, the marginals, the non-productive, and in general those who caused a crisis in the family and social order through the exhibition of their suffering.

Entering an asylum meant the civil death of the inpatients, not only because they were deprived of their capacity to exert the normal civil rights but also because, through the ritual of undressing, they were deprived of all their personal objects. As in prison, these objects were put in a sealed bag that could be open only on the day of discharge—something that rarely happened. This meant to deprive them of their social identity by interrupting every significant relationship with the outside world.

Concentration camps saw the loss of the desire to live due to the daily attacks on dignity and self-esteem, on people's sense of mastery and self-control, on their physical integrity—that is, on the entire narcissism of the human being. The same can be said of people who spent their entire existence in an asylum.

The institutionalised person withers in the lack of interests: he has inside himself a desert that instinctually pushes, or a vegetative life slowly moves (De Vincentiis, 1979).

Today it is still possible to hear many relatives of inpatients speak of them as having passed away, as if they were dead, as if it only those events before they were hospitalised are worth remembering, as if the image of death were consumed in advance. Public discourse uses the metaphor of travel to refer to a departure without a return from another world for both the dying (a journey to the afterlife) and the psychiatric patients (a journey to the world of madness) (Giroletti, 1996).

The most significant expression of this clandestine state and anonymity can be found in the cemetery of the village near the psychiatric hospital of Cogoleto.

The section of the Nativity Scene dedicated to the cemetery near the asylum (Figure 11.1) allows the viewer to immediately perceive the

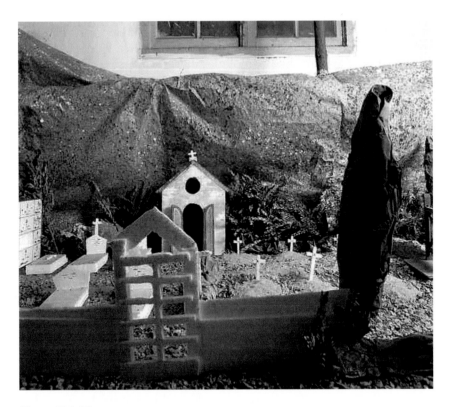

Figure 11.1 The cemetery.

difference between the field where the fools are buried and the one where those who did not die in the asylum are buried. They are neatly distinguished: in the former there is a set of identical crosses transmitting the sense of uniformity, massification, anonymity; the latter lacks this sad egalitarianism and the tombs have different size, shape, style, economical value according to class, social relevance, and the belonging culture of the dead. Even when dead, the fools remain anonymous: once they dressed in the same uniforms; now they have the same tombs. Because of this absence of individuality, they are interchangeable.

According to Papi (1980), the cemetery is the social and meeting place of the public and the private because of the distinction between the living and the dead. Everyone is here, in an almost clear expression of the fact that, once dead, no one has the social role that they played when alive. However, Papi's considerations lose their value when a cemetery must include the corpses of the inpatients of a psychiatric hospital. Not even death, which many buried alive considered a liberation, allows equality, as Totò (De Curtis A.) (1989) writes in his poem "'A livella" ("The level").

Even today, a hilly road definitively divides the cemetery of Cogoleto in two sectors: above the "normal" dead, below the dead of the asylum who were buried at night so as not to disturb or create a scandal, as shown in the part of the Nativity Scene in which a nurse moves a corpse on a wooden cart, like a smuggler illegally crossing the border of the world of madmen (Figure 11.2). Immediately one can notice in the upstream field the movement determined by the presence of tombs of different shapes, sizes, and colours, representing different expressions of condolences, which in turn reflect cultural, economic, and social differences.

Given that everyone has their grave, the simulacrum of identity remains.

The stereotyped pictures and the funeral dedications indicate an attempt to seek an individuation of the dead and bestow upon them ancient recognition.

In the field down the road a tidy flattening can be immediately perceived: it is a succession of equal rows of memorials of common stone, each one having painted a number by hand. It is a dry summary of a non-life, which time has faded away first and completely cancelled later, thus making impossible any chance of identification. Dead without names, memory, history; unworthy dead, scandalous dead, unrecognisable dead.

In the 1970s the memorials were reconstructed in marble. Brass plates were affixed, stating the names and dates of birth and death. However, the visual sensation of anonymity has not disappeared, only attenuated. Only in recent years, thanks to the possibility of using their money deposited in the hospital's finance offices, some patients could have paid a funeral, a decent coffin, and a recognisable tomb.

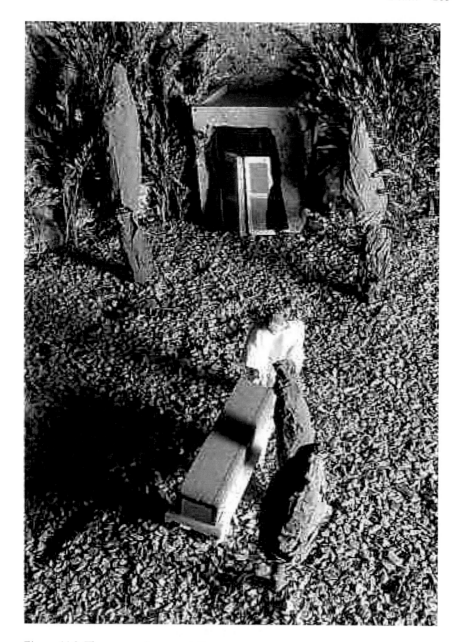

Figure 11.2 The corpse transportation.

Unfortunately, the sectors reserved for the asylum inpatients are still physically separated from the other ones. Deep phobic anxieties of contagion, aiming to avoid any contact with the stranger, determine these absurd and gross operations of separations. A neat separation, a sort of *postmortem* barrier, gives some respectability to the living. The place of the dead, all resting in peace in the "right soil," works like a family tree. This is the heritage of Medieval norms, although traceable in marginalised funerary practices, for which the fools should be buried in a desecrated soil like suicide victims.

Death in a psychiatric hospital is something clandestine for those who live outside the institution. No visible sign of it is given, no burial announcements, no funeral ritual symbols. Nonetheless, death is not hidden inside the institution: it is cynically exhibited as something without any social value or symbolic meaning. Public indifference accompanies this state.

If the inpatient was considered already dead at the social level when he entered the asylum, then his physical death is nothing but a detail, an annoying appendix of a just written and announced event. The presence of the dead does not touch the daily routine of the asylum in any manner.

If the inpatient dies at night, then his body remains in the bed until the next day, in direct contact with the other roommates. At best, when a nurse notices the corpse, he covers it with a sheer. Some old patients report that until the 1960s the dormitories were so big and full that often deaths were not noticed until after much time passed. Almost always, patients remained silent and apathetic, showing a chronic confusion between death and institutional life.

The disappearance of someone did not call for commentary. There was no involved or resigned sharing of the event because isolation did not become discretion or social dignity. Rather, it was a serious instance of undifferentiation and mixing, cancelling every symbolic connotation of the dead body and eliminating its every significant feature.

In the asylum privacy is not a value: the lewd exhibition of the corpse is the triumph of cynicism, indifference, anonymity, apathy, strangeness, and impassiveness.

Life autonomously flows and touches the organic structures, only animating the metabolic factors and erasing that exclusive human skill of living our death and that of the others.

That thin veil spread over the truth of death, that discrete and fearful not talking about it, are replaced by a clear, clean, detached, and icy pronunciation of death (Schinaia and Molteni, 1986).

Even the ritual of the so-called religious comfort occurs hastily and confidentially.

When children die in paediatric wards, they are dressed in the most beautiful clothes and, most of the time, in general hospitals relatives are asked to dress the dead patients with clean and decorous clothes. Meanwhile, in the asylum, the ritual dressing of the dead simply does not exist (Schinaia, 1983, 2023a). In fact, the dead were dressed in the so-called death shirt, a large white shirt with a faded cross sewn above. The death shirt was taken away when the corpse was put naked into the coffin, which consisted of four grossly nailed boards, so that it could be used afterwards.

In contrast to what happens in the wards of a general hospital, especially in the paediatric ones, physicians and nurses are not emotionally involved, acting out massive and gross defence mechanisms. When present, the relatives are indifferent or relieved. When they arrive at the asylum, everything has just happened in solitude, without the hypothetical comfort of their presence.

Cynicism, absence of affectivity, relational degradation, and flattening of the mourning expression are the final points of an exclusion process begun when the patient entered the asylum.

Recovering the private rituality and reproposing the mourning as a social and psychological necessity can be the basis for a renewed respect of the dying and the dead, in every place and manner he dies. This demands that we effectively pay attention to individuation in contrast to anonymity and that solitude exist without piety and commiseration. This could be achieved with the elimination of those institutional places of exclusion such as the psychiatric hospital. All this depends on our willingness to include, once again, in social circles the scandalous death of the fool.

12   Between Past and Future

Most women and men held in the Psychiatric Hospital of Cogoleto experienced a form of social and affective displacement similar to exile.

They felt in their bodies and minds the pain of the house falling apart that Primo Levi describes in *Survival in Auschwitz* (1947), in which he invites the reader to imagine a person deprived of everyone she or he loves and, at the same time, of her or his house, habits, clothes, and everything she or he possesses. The result can be only a hollow person reduced to suffering and basic needs, without dignity and restraint, for he or she who loses all, easily loses himself or herself.

The patients were taken away from their homes and environments: they had to leave the countryside or the cities where they lived and were put in an isolated and remote place, whose norms, language, and institutional functioning were unknown and totally alienated from their direct experience and even more from their control. They were forced to be in a precarious condition and therefore to continuously desire safe landmarks. It is something similar to what Calvino describes in *Invisible Cities* (1972), writing of different cities that follow one another in the same place and under the same name, born and dying without knowing each other, without communicating.

Habit and inhabiting have the same etymological root. To emigrate is to change habits. One feels anxious, perplexed, and unsafe. If we think about living in an asylum, we quickly realise that it is practically impossible to find protection or safety there. The institutionalised space of the hospital is the denial of the protective home space in which we can move with the certainty of what surrounds us. That is a space containing and safeguarding us. Without such protective qualities, not only spatial but also temporal and vital movements become impossible. Not being at home provokes anxiety, feelings of disorientation, of being lost, that is, of being in an indeterminate place, in nothing, in nowhere.

The farewell guarantees a protective framework to the border crossed when one leaves. The ritual provides virtual signals to what is elusive: these signals are like a compass tracing a horizon in critical moments (Grinberg and Grinberg, 1984). The exiled cannot have the farewell ritual.

DOI: 10.4324/9781003381723-12

This is the same (and perhaps more significant) for the future inhabitants of the asylum: they are deprived of the social and affective container of the abandonment anxiety and desperation for their losses. The missed farewell ceremony is added to their anxieties, so that departure is experienced as crossing the border between the realm of the living and the realm of the dead. One of the defence mechanisms against separation anxiety and contact with the unknown and mysterious world of the asylum is to deny the present. The present time remains squeezed between the transfigured and mythicised past life and the future life represented by the impossible hope to return to the fantasised and not realistic place of origin. An Ego failing to deal with the mourning mechanism can lead to the traumatic loss of an object. This loss can later provoke a reduction of the will to work through the mourning (Kleiner, 1970). This can be seen when the institutionalised patient appears detached, cynical, even mocking of a rehabilitative project providing the chance to realistically confront the external world.

De Martis (1995) points out that some patients show a surprising clairvoyance, allowing them to readily understand the intention of an interlocutor. Such a clairvoyance emerges from the abyss of radical indifference and arrogant distance they use to immunise themselves from long-term suffering. It is an invitation expressed in a strong *noli me tangere* (do not touch me). The old psychiatry interpreted this discouraging invitation as athymia. Perhaps the most relevant discovery of psycho-analytic psychotherapy was to recognise in patients an intense demand for communication despite their legitimate diffidence. In good relational conditions, this demand can become a transference, frail and lukewarm at first, then passionate and overwhelming.

The misery of daily reality and the grandeur of the past cannot be compared. The patient talks about things that for the therapist are in another time and space but that for them are so present and recognisable that the therapist is totally excluded (Sohn, 1983).

Nostalgia transforms into regret for a past and for significant but irre-cuperable people because there was a fracture between a love object of the present, that had lost life and splendour, and the relationships of the past that, as internal objects, are idealised.

A typical trait of nostalgia is that absence, hiatus, and loss acquire so high a value that they become idealised and magnified (Petrella, 1993g).

Although a place is not only a physical place but also the words and events inhabiting it, it is nevertheless around its denied visibility, around its disappearance from the sight, that we feel nostalgia (Prete, 1992).

Autistic isolation can be a challenge to the inacceptable institutional routine, a response to its Kafkian nonsense, a sublimation of the absence of contacts and relationships, a monument to the memory of something that cannot be recovered. Autism can be the theatrical representation of the exasperation of solitude and nostalgia. But, at the same time, losing every link with original feelings, it has its own dimension strongly boosted and defined by institutional logos, which cancels every meaning that cannot be explained in its intrinsic logic.

The construction of the Nativity Scene filled the void of an idealised absence with the history of the institution, a history mainly of pain and violence but also of friendships, affects, minimal forms of solidarity, and social recognition (the café, the theatre, the workplaces). The birthplace was inhospitable and expulsive but became a fantastic original place in contrast to the image of an institutional past life. Building projects of transformation can only be possible by changing this idealised image and replacing it with a hard and not consolatory representation of institutional life, thus showing all its contradictions. Under such conditions, these projects must be based on historical context, not ideological prejudice.

However, the construction of the Nativity Scene could support regression and nostalgia. In fact, art can be both a source of anxiety and what neutralises it by showing, as museums do, institutional reality, something without a proposal to go beyond it. The hospital's farm could become a bucolic ideal instead of a place of exploitation; its school could look like the school of our memories, the brutal images of the wards' interiors could refer to a painful order in contrast with a disorganised and unpoetic present.

The observer is lost in this nostalgic perspective in a labyrinth of a sort of past beauty. The vanity of regret and the movements of remembrance idealise the institutional past, devalue the present, and devitalise the future.

According to Petrella (1993g), the object of nostalgia is something desired or absent containing the promise of happiness that can minimise or damage the value of the present and available object. Thus, the present object is not significant in comparison with the past object. The present object does not correspond to the ideal one and thus has no real value. Rather, the past object, which desire obstinately turns into something nostalgic, is either inaccessible or no longer desirable, at least not in its present form.

The view of Genoa (Figure 12.1), the big and ideal city, alludes to a place in which human beings can find themselves again and integrate with others (Meriana, 1996). Its houses go from the sea to the mountains, the salty sea consuming the soft-pastel hues of their façades. It is a beautiful and moving image, but it is a nostalgic outlook. As Calvino (1972) points out, every city is shaped from the desert it opposes.

Most patients came from Genoa, but the Genoa of the Nativity Scene is a splendid city coming from the deceiving transfiguration of memory, not the beginning of the long path of suffering and exclusion. In fact, most inpatients came from the greyish degraded suburbs or from the ruined hovels of the historic city centre.

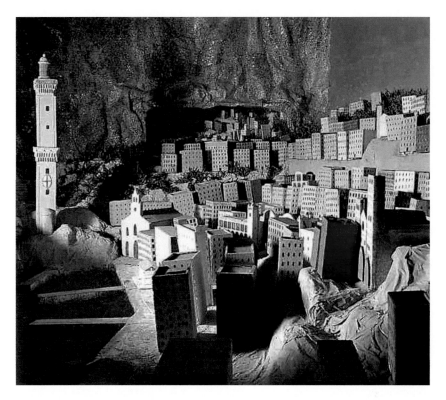

Figure 12.1 View of Genoa.

For many of them, the anonymous dormitories/buildings without any colour or community represented the last stop on a journey started in a sunny town of Southern Italy. Emigration deeply destroys the collective mechanisms of regulation of the critical moments of existence. These mechanisms are particularly active in societies from which the migration flows begin. It follows that the feeling of lack of protection related to the traumatic experience of emigration coincides with the experience of the loss of the container (Bion, 1970). In extreme cases, this leads to the disintegration and dissolution of the Ego and the loss of its borders. This is more strongly felt if childhood has been characterised by significant experiences of deprivation and separation and their related feelings of anxiety and lack of protection (Grinberg and Grinberg, 1984).

The nostalgic transfiguration makes Genoa unreachable, an unrealisable hypothesis, a dream contrasting with the unavoidable and unchangeable misery of the asylum's daily routine.

In contrast, another scene shows the project, the future, the hope based on something concrete. It is the scene in which the spectator can have an overall view of the sea, the town of Cogoleto, and the hill where the

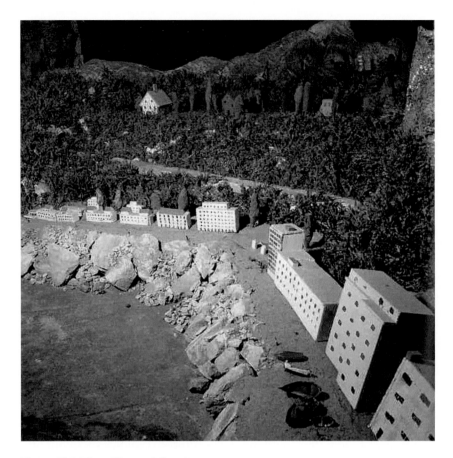

Figure 12.2 The village of Cogoleto.

asylum stands (Figure 12.2). Here both the break of separation and integration are possible and reachable. There is something new, vital, and transformative. In fact, the town of Cogoleto is not far from the asylum; it can be reached. It represents the first step of a realistic return to Genoa. It is the possibility of a journey using new maps. Going beyond agoraphobia is possible thanks to a project respecting both the potential and limitations, without granting anything to the regressive and comforting claustrophilia. The image of Genoa at the end of the journey is a mix of open contradictions, a pulsating and vital conglomerate in contrast with the timeless and deadly air of the asylum.

The nostalgic emotion is both caesura and suture with the past and, re-proposed in the present space of the narrative, seems to refer to the future change like the water of a stream that flows into other ones and seems to be looking for a new riverbed (Gaburri, 1989). The risk shared not only by the patients but also by the physicians and nurses is to look for comfort in "the way we were," distorted by the difficulties of imagining a realisable future. They have fantasies of living in a separate world that cannot be shared with others and in which the usual temporal parameters are suspended. It is a matter of coming to terms with a present full of difficulties but situated in a field where chronicity is in touch with the time of collective life, work, exchanges, and passions.

According to Correale (1991), accepting the temporal dimension is a crucial achievement for every human being. Thinking of the past and future inevitably creates in chronic patients not only dismay but also the painful feeling of coming to terms with themselves, finding inside themselves hated and feared scenarios, abhorred and terrifying ghosts.

The projects to go beyond the idea of asylum can start from these reflections. These projects must be thought out and realised not only in terms of sophisticated architectural and procedural operations (which are mandatory, of course) but also in terms of attempts to construct a livability compatible with the surrounding social environment.

The surrounding environment and habitat must be thought out more in psychological than in spatial terms; that is, as physical and mental collective places able to accept and contain that ineludible eccentricity and radical diversity of the psychotic, of the Other as someone different but not a stranger.

Afterword by Giovanna Rotondi Terminiello

I first visited the place that housed the Cogoleto "Other Nativity Scene," as Dr. Cosimo Schinaia called it in the first Italian edition of his book, in 1995. This unique piece of artwork thanks to a collective creativity had already existed for about 15 years. Its main creators, the artist Bruno Galati (the creator of most of the puppets and scenography of the Nativity Scene) and the nurse Tomaso Molinari (perhaps the main promoter of this artwork inside the hospital), had continuously monitored it and tended to it with repairs and regular maintenance. Thus, I found it still well preserved.

When Cosimo Schinaia asked me to inspect the site of the psychiatric hospital, I was Superintendent of Archaeology, Fine Arts and Landscape for Liguria and thus responsible for its artistic heritage. I was surprised by a totally unexpected vision: I had expected to see a traditional nativity scene. I felt an increasing apprehension walking through that tortuous corridor with the scenes lining the walls. I was immediately aware of the exceptional character of this work thanks to its connections to the history of psychiatric hospitals. It was a dramatic collective testimony of a public institution at the beginning of its dismantling.

I immediately assessed the risks of survival of the Nativity Scene if it did not have continuous care after the closure of the hospital. Some endemic factors of the nature of conservation justified my worries: the instable thermohygrometric conditions, worsened by the lack of air intake in the space; the very frail and degradable materials used for the Nativity Scene (paper, cardboard, papier-mâché, polystyrene, rags, branches, dry leaves, etc.); the consequences of the presence of rodents because the ground floor location, in a wooded environment, of the corridor used for setting up the Nativity Scene.

I was unable to limit these dangers from a legal perspective: the law for the protection of artistic and historical interests excluded work carried out less than 50 years before. Therefore, the possibilities of legal protection of the "Other Nativity Scene" were only foreseeable in the future, not before 2030 or, in other terms, after the highly likely collapse of the work!

Furthermore, all the calls for conservative vigilance, with their appeal to the collective sense of responsibility, were in vain so that the decline of the artwork soon became evident. The first official statement of degradation and marginalisation came in 2007.

Today, after about 16 years, the damage has increased in geometric progression and led to some irreparable consequences.

So, what is the future of the Other Nativity Scene?

It is hoped that the place in which the Nativity Scene will be hosted will not be completely different from the original context in which it was created.

However, I ask myself if such an operation can be consistent with what the creators of the Nativity Scene wanted, thought, and did because of an urgent disillusion and aimed to express their diversity from other people. From here followed the choice to set aside traditional execution techniques and use degradable materials, coherent with the realisation of an artwork representing yesterday's today, a "today" left at the mercy of time and a transient life path.

It is, of course, certain that, whatever the future of the Nativity Scene, its memory is already fixed thanks to its ample photographic documentation throughout the years and the rich bibliography that, starting from the research of Cosimo Schinaia, will continue to remember it, at least in the world of science.

References

Accornero, A. (1980). *Il Lavoro come Ideologia*. Bologna: Il Mulino.

Alberti, L.B. (1452). *On the Art of Building in Ten Books*. J. Rykwert, R. Tavernor, and N. Leach (Trans.). Washington: Library of the Congress, 1988.

American Psychiatric Association (1989). *Treatments of Psychiatric Disorders. A Task Force Report of the American Psychiatric Association, Vol. 3*. Washington: American Psychiatric Association.

American Psychiatric Association (1990). The Practice of ECT. Recommendations for Treatment, Research and Training. *Convulsive Therapy*, 6(2): 85–120.

Ammaniti, M. (1995). *"Maternal Care and Mental Health,"* di Bowlby a 40 Anni dalla Sua Pubblicazione: I Nuovi Paradigmi in Campo Infantile. *Prospettive Psicoanalitiche nel Lavoro Istituzionale*, 13(1): 35–45.

Anonymous (1909). *Lettera dei medici di Quarto al Mare alla Deputazione Provinciale. Quarto al Mare, 28/4/1909* Archivio storico della Provincia di Genova, Categoria VII, Assistenza pubblica: Manicomi, b. 20, fasc. 9.

Ariès, Ph. (1974). *Western Attitudes toward Death: From the Middle Ages to the Present*. P.M. Ranum (Trans.). Baltimore: Johns Hopkins University Press.

Ariès, Ph. (1977). *The Hour of Our Death*. H. Weaver (Trans.). London: Penguin Books, 1983.

Asioli, F., Ballerini, A., and Berti Ceroni, G. (Eds.) (1993). *Psichiatria nella Comunità*. Turin: Bollati Boringhieri.

Azzurri, F. (1877). Intervento al II° Congresso della Società Freniatrica Italiana (Aversa). *Archivio Italiano per le Malattie Nervose e Più Particolarmente per le Alienazioni Mentali*: 427–428.

Babini, V.P., Cotti, M., Minuz, F., and Tagliavini, A. (1982). *Tra Sapere e Potere. La Psichiatria Italiana nella Seconda Metà dell'Ottocento*. Bologna: Il Mulino.

Bakwin, H. (1942). Loneliness in Infants. *American Journal of Diseases in Children*, 63(1): 30–40.

Balbo, P.P. (1993). Per una Ridefinizione del Concetto di Piazza. In: A. Marino (Ed.), op. cit. (pp. 214–216).

Balduzzi, E. (1962). *Le Terapie di Shock*. Milan: Feltrinelli.

Balduzzi, E. (1969). L'Assistenza nella Schizofrenia Cronica. *Aut Aut*, 113: 57–77.

Balduzzi, E. (1989). Les Coopératives. Instruments de Réhabilitation. *L'Information Psychiatrique*, 7: 722–725.

Barale, F. (1982). Lutto, Funzione Simbolica e Atteggiamento Medico verso il Morente. *Archivio di Psicologia, Neurologia e Psichiatria*, 2: 254–265.

Barisone, M., and Schinaia, C. (1995). Rianimazione Istituzionale e Alfabetizzazione nel Lavoro con Psicotici Cronici. In: P.M. Furlan (Ed.), op. cit. (pp. 183–190).

Barthes, R. (1973). *The Pleasure of the Text*. R. Miller (Trans.). New York: Hill and Wang, 1975.

Basaglia, F. (1981–1982). *Scritti, 2 Vol*. Turin: Einaudi.

Basaglia, F., Scheper-Hughes, N., and Lovell, A.M. (Eds.) (1987). *Psychiatry Inside Out: Selected Writings of Franco Basaglia*. T. Shtob (Trans.). New York: Columbia University Press.

Bellonzi, M. (2016). Il Primo Ballo all'Ospedale di Bonifazio. La Psichiatria Innovativa di Francesco Bini. Fondazione Santa Maria Nuova. http://www.fondazionesantamarianuova.com/contents/il-primo-ballo-allospedale-di-bonifazio.

Bender, L. (1947). Psychopathic Behaviors Disorder in Children. In: R.M. Lindner and R.V. Seliger (Eds.), op. cit., (pp. 360–377).

Benevelli, L. (1996). Ergoterapia, Lavoro, Occupazione: I Servizi di Salute Mentale e il Diritto al Lavoro. *Fogli di Informazione*, 168: 28–40.

Berger, M. (1978). Formation aux Soins aux Mourants. *Perspectives Psychiatriques*, 66: 133–138.

Berke, J. (1972). ECT: The Slaughterhouse Discovery. *General Practitioner*, April.

Bertelli, C. and G. Bollati, G. (Eds.) (1979). Storia d'Italia. Annali 2. *L'Immagine Fotografica 1845–1945*. Turin: Einaudi.

Bertolini, A., and Casarino, L. (1974). Contributo all'Analisi della Problematica Connessa con l'Uso dell'Elettroshockterapia. *Neuropsichiatria*, 30 (3–4): 317–330.

Bettanini, A., and Moreno, D. (1970). *Il Presepe Genovese*. Genoa: Sagep.

Bion, W.R. (1962). *Learning from Experience*. New York: Aronson, 1994.

Bion, W.R. (1970). *Attention and Interpretation*. London and New York: Routledge.

Boatti, G. (2012). *Sulle Strade del Silenzio. Viaggio per Monasteri d'Italia e Spaesati Dintorni*. Rome-Bari: Laterza.

Bollati, G. (1979). Note su Fotografia e Storia. In: C. Bertelli and G. Bollati (Eds.), op. cit., (pp. 3–55). Turin: Einaudi.

Bollorino F. and Valdrè, R. (Eds.) (1996). Il Caso Buttolo. *Una Cartella Clinica d'Inizio Secolo*. Turin: UTET.

Bordi, M., Boccianti, N., Bersani, I., and Risso, M.D. (1995). Psicosi e Lavoro: Richiesta Impossibile o Illusione Che Cura?. *Il Vaso di Pandora*, III(4): 153–156.

Bordignon Elestici, L. (1991). *Presepi nel Mondo. Itinerari d'Immagini*. Milan: BE-MA Editrice.

Borges, J., and Bioy Casares, A. (1967). *Chronicles of Bustos-Domecq*. N.T. Di Giovanni (Trans.). New York: Dutton, 1979.

Borrelli, G. (1991). *Il Presepe Napoletano*. Naples: Pironti.

Bosazzi, P., and Venezia, S. (1986). Il Presepe. Storia di follia. *Liguria Medica*, 11: 23–27.

Bowlby, J. (1951). Maternal Care and Mental Health. *Bulletin of the World Health Organization*, 3: 355–533.

Breggin, P.R. (1979). *Electroshock, Its Brain-Disabling Effects*. New York: Springer.

Breggin, P.R., and De Girolamo, G. (1987). Elettroshock: Tra Rischio Iatrogeno e Mito Terapeutico. *Quaderni Italiani di Psichiatria*, 6: 497–540.

Buoniconti Aschettino, A. (1992). Il Presepe nelle Varie Regioni d'Italia: Tradizione, Diffusione, Varietà di Concezione. *Il Presepio*, 150: 19–22.

Burlingham, D., and Freud, A. (1943). *Infants without Families*. London: Allen and Unwin.

Buzzati, D. (1940). *The Tartar Steppe*. S.C. Hood (Trans.). London: Secker and Warburg, 1952.

Calvino, I. (1972). *Invisible Cities*. W. Weaver (Trans.). London: Vintage, 1997.

Calvino, I. (1983). Accanto a una Mostra. *FMR, July–August, 15:* 40–52.

Canosa, R. (1979). *Storia del Manicomio in Italia dall'Unità a Oggi.* Milan: Feltrinelli.

Capuano, M. (Ed.) (2009). Miss Architect. Architetture al Femminile. Architettonicamente. Pisa: ETS.

Carloni, G. (1984). Il Trauma della Nascita e la Nascita di una Rivista. *Rivista di Psicoanalisi, 30*(4): 494–508.

Carloni, G. (1989). Tragitti della Nostalgia. In: S. Vecchio (Ed.), op. cit. (pp. 119–129).

Carpaneto, C. (1953). *Pammatone. Cinque Secoli di Vita Ospedaliera.* Genoa: Ospedali Civili.

Cassirer, E. (1944). *An Essay on Man: An Introduction to a Philosophy of Human Culture.* New Haven: Yale University Press.

Castel, R. (1976), L'Ordine Psichiatrico. L'Epoca d'Oro dell'Alienismo. G. Procacci (It. Trans.). Milan: Feltrinelli, 1980. En. translation: Castel, R. (1976). The Regulation of Madness. The Origins of Incarceration in France. W.D. Halls (Trans.). Berkeley, CA: University of California Press, 1988.

Catalano Nobili, C. and Cerquetelli, G. (1972). *L'Elettroshock.* Rome: Il Pensiero Scientifico.

Cataldi Gallo, M. (1993). La Moda in Miniatura. In: Soprintendenza per i Beni Artistici e Storici della Liguria (Ed.), op. cit. (pp. 74–83).

Causa, R. (1987). La Stagione Aurea del Presepe Napoletano. In: M. Piccoli Catello (Ed.), op. cit., (pp. 19–33).

Cerati, G. (Ed.) (1993). *La Fantasia al Lavoro.* Turin: Bollati Boringhieri.

Cerletti, U., and Bini, L. (1938). L'Elettroshock. *Archivio Generale di Neurologia, Psichiatria, Psicoanalisi, 19:* 266–268.

Cerletti, U. (1950). Old and New Information about Electroshock. *American Journal of Psychiatry, 107:* 87–94.

Cervellini, F. (1993). La Piazza È Morta. Viva la Piazza. In: A. Marino (Ed.), op. cit. (pp. 212–214).

C.G.I.L., C.I.S.L., U.I.L (1974). *Libro Bianco sui Manicomi Genovesi.* Genoa: A.T.A.

Chekhov, A. (1892). *Ward No. 6 and Other Stories, 1892–1895.* R. Wilks (Ed. and Trans.). London: Penguin, 2002.

Ciancaglini, P., Russano, M., and Schinaia, C. (1989). Lo Psicotico e la Sua Casa. Riflessioni sul Ruolo dell'Abitazione del Paziente Psicotico nella Relazione Terapeutica. In: F. Petrella (Ed.), op. cit. (pp. 121–128).

Cianconi P. (2013). Teoria dell'Interstizio e Psicopatologia. *Psichiatria Oggi, 4, XV:* 1–3.

Citati, P. (1997). Perché Ci Piace Ancora il Presepe. *La Repubblica,* January 2.

Coffey, C.E., and Weiner, R.D. (1990). Electroconvulsive Therapy: An Update. *Hospital & Community Psychiatry, 41:* 515–521.

Colafelice, M. (1993). L'Inserimento Lavorativo dei Pazienti Psichiatrici. *Rivista di Riabilitazione Psichiatrica e Psicosociale, 2*(2): 87–91.

Comitato Nazionale per la Bioetica (1996). Parere sull'Eticità della Terapia Elettroconvulsivante del 1995. *Medicina e Morale, 4:* 796–801.

Conforto, C. (1996). Una Chiave di Lettura Psicoanalitica. In: F. Bollorino and R. Valdrè (Eds.), op. cit., (pp. 213–222).

Corradi Fiumara, G. (1980). *Funzione Simbolica e Filosofia del Linguaggio.* Turin: Boringhieri.

Correale, A. (1991). *Il Campo Istituzionale.* Rome: Borla.

Crepet, P., and Righetti, A. (1985). Elettroshock?. *Psicoterapia e Scienze Umane*, *19*(2): 59–73.

Crepet, P. (1990). *Le Malattie della Disoccupazione*. Rome: Edizioni del Lavoro.

Cristicchi, S. (2007). *Centro di Igiene Mentale. Un Cantastorie tra i Matti*. Milan: Mondadori.

Dartington, T., Menzies Lyth, I., and Williams Polacco, G.W. (1992). *Bambini in Ospedale. Una Ricerca della Tavistock Clinic*. R. Schapiter, M.J. Petrone, and P. Fabozzi (Trans.). Naples: Liguori. Italian translation of *The Psychological Welfare of Young Children Making Long Stays in Hospital. Final Report*. Tavistock Institute of Human Relations, Doc. No. CASR 1200.

De Bernardi, A., De Peri, F., and Panzeri, L. (1980). *Tempo e Catene. Manicomio, Psichiatria e Classi Subalterne. Il Caso Milanese*. Milan: FrancoAngeli.

De Frémenville, B. (1977). *La Raison du Plus Fort. Traiter ou Maltraiter les Fous?* Paris: Seuil.

De Giacomo, U. (1960). *L'Assistenza Psichiatrica Odierna. Nozioni per il Personale di Vigilanza negli Ospedali Psichiatrici*. Rome: Edizioni Mediterranee.

De Girolamo, G. (1993). L'Elettroshock: Una Rassegna Critica. In: F. Asioli, A. Ballerini, and G. Berti Ceroni (Eds.), op. cit. (pp. 407–417).

De Intinis, G. (Ed.) (2023). *Quaderno di Psicoanalisi e Sociale*. Rome: Vecchiarelli.

De Leeuw, R. (Ed.) (1996). *The Letters of Vincent van Gogh*, A.J. Pomerans (Trans.). London: Penguin.

De Leonardis, O., Mauri, D. and Rotelli, F. (1994). *L'Impresa Sociale*. Milan: Anabasi.

De Leonardis, O., and Emmenegger, T. (2005). Le Istituzioni della Contraddizione. *Rivista Sperimentale di Freniatria*, 3: 7–33.

De Martis, D. (1987). L'Assistenza Psichiatrica: Un Antico Problema Sempre di Attualità nella Pubblica Opinione. In: D. De Martis et al. (Eds.), op. cit. (pp. 7–17).

De Martis, D. (1995). Cronicità e Psicoterapia. In: P.M. Furlan (Ed.), op. cit. (pp. 3–7).

De Martis, D., Petrella, F., and Caverzasi, E. (Eds.) (1980). *Il Paese degli Specchi*. Milan: Feltrinelli.

De Martis, D., Petrella, F., and Ambrosi, P. (Eds.) (1987). *La Riforma Psichiatrica: Il Linguaggio dei Quotidiani. Un'Indagine e una Riflessione Critica*. Milan: FrancoAngeli.

De Peri, F. (1984). Il Medico e il Folle: Istituzione Psichiatrica, Sapere Scientifico e Pensiero Medico fra Otto e Novecento. In: F. Della Peruta (Ed.), op. cit., (pp. 1057–1140).

De Salvia, D. (1977). *Per una Psichiatria Alternativa*. Milan: Feltrinelli.

De Vincentiis, G. (1979). La Cultura della Morte e il Mondo dell'Istituzionalizzazione. *Rivista Sperimentale di Freniatria*, 103: 261–298.

Della Peruta, F. (Ed.) (1984). Storia d'Italia. *Annali 7*. Turin: Einaudi.

Di Chiara, G. (1979). La Psicoanalisi e la Separazione, Prefazione. In: P. Ferrari (Ed.), op. cit., (pp. XI–XXI).

Di Chiara, G. (1994). È Possibile Individuare i Fattori che Promuovono la Buona Relazione? In: A. Ferruta et al. (Eds.), op. cit. (pp. 197–216).

Direzione dei "Quaderni di Psichiatria" (1917). Il Lavoro degli Anormali Psichici e la Guerra. *Quaderni di Psichiatria*, 4: 79–83.

Dörner, K. (1969). Il Borghese e il Folle. F. Giacanelli and M.C. Boriosi (It. Trans.). Rome-Bari: Laterza, 1975.

Dostoevsky, F. (1864). *Notes from Underground*, R. Pevear and L. Volokhonsky (Trans.). London: Vintage, 1994.

Duby, G. (1973). *Early Growth of the European Economy: Warriors and Peasants from the Seventh to the Twelfth Century.* H.B. Clarke (Trans.). Ithaca, New York: Cornell University Press, 1978.

Esquirol, J.-E.-D. (1838). *Mental Maladies: A Treatise on Insanity,* E.K. Hunt (Trans.). Philadelphia: Lea and Blanchard, 1845.

Fenichel, O. (1945). *The Psychoanalytic Theory of Neurosis.* London and New York: Routledge, 1996.

Ferenczi, S. (1949). Confusion of Tongues between Adults and the Child: The Language of Tenderness and the Language of Passion. *International Journal of Psycho-Analysis, 30*: 225–230.

Ferrari, P. (Ed.) (1976). *Le Separazioni dalla Nascita alla Morte.* S. Rossi (It. Trans.). Rome: Il Pensiero Scientifico, 1979.

Ferro, F.M. (1979). L'Uso dei Farmaci Non Deve Andare oltre Piccole Dosi. *Fogli di Informazione, 57/58*: 373–375.

Ferro, F.M., Gaddini, A., and Riefolo, G. (1995). Del Buon Uso delle Cose nella Terapia della Cronicità. In: P.M. Furlan (Ed.), op.cit. (pp. 485–493).

Ferro, M., Maccioni, L., and Schinaia, C. (1993). Il Comprensorio Terapeutico Riabilitativo. *Prospettive Sociali e Sanitarie, 17*: 18–20.

Ferruta, A., Galli, T. and Lojacono, N. (Eds.) (1994). Uno Spazio Condiviso. La terapia dei pazienti psicotici in una struttura intermedia. Rome: Borla.

Ferruta, A. (2009). Architetture della Mente. In: M. Capuano (Ed.), op. cit., (pp. 22–26).

Flesher, J. (1949). Further Contributions to the Psychodynamics of Convulsive Treatment. *Journal of Nervous and Mental Disease, 109*: 550–554.

Fodor, N. (1950). Varieties of Nostalgia. *Psychoanalytic Review, 37*: 25–38.

Fornari, F. (1976). *Simbolo e Codice.* Milan: Feltrinelli.

Fornari, F. (1981). *Il Codice Vivente.* Turin: Boringhieri.

Freud, S. (1893). Charcot. *S.E., 3*: 7–23.

Freud, S. (1907). Delusion and Dream in Jensen's Gradiva. *S.E., 9*: 7–95.

Freud, S. (1909). Family Romances. *S.E., 9*: 237–241.

Freud, S. (1913 [1912–13]). Totem and Taboo: Some Points of Agreement between the Mental Lives of Savages and Neurotics. In: Totem and Taboo and Other Works (1913–1914). *S.E., 13*: vii–162.

Freud, S. (1915). Thoughts for the Times on War and Death. *S.E., 14*: 289–300.

Freud, S. (1917). Mourning and Melancholia. *S.E., 14*: 237–258.

Freud, S. (1920a). Memorandum on the Electrical Treatment of War Neurotics. *S.E., 17*: 211–215.

Freud, S. (1920b). Beyond the Pleasure Principle. *S.E., 18*: 1–64.

Freud, S. (1926). Inhibitions, Symptoms and Anxiety. *S.E., 20*: 87–174.

Freud, S. (1930). Civilisation and Its Discontents. *S.E., 21*: 59–145.

Freud, S. (1933). New Introductory Lectures on Psycho-Analysis. *S.E., 22*: 1–182.

Fuchs, W. (1969). *Le Immagini della Morte nella Società Moderna.* G. Dore (It. Trans.). Turin: Einaudi, 1973.

Furlan, P.M. (Ed.) (1995). *Psicoterapia e Cronicità.* Turin: CST.

Gaburri, E. (1989). La Partenza da Ogigia, ovvero della Nostalgia. In: S. Vecchio (Ed.), op. cit. (pp. 143–149).

Gaburri, E. (1994). Piero Leonardi: Uno Psicoanalista nell'Istituzione Psichiatrica. *Rivista di Psicoanalisi, 40*(2): 345–354.

Gadda, C.E. (1961). *That Awful Mess on Via Merulana.* W. Weaver (Trans.). New York: Review Books Classics, 2007.

Gaddini, E. (1984). Changes in Psychoanalytic Patients Up to the Present Day. In: E. Gaddini and A. Limentani (Eds.), *A Psychoanalytic Theory of Infantile Experience: Conceptual and Clinic Reflections* (pp. 195–203). London and New York: Routledge, 1992.

Gaddini, E. (1985). La Nascita, la Crescita. In: Id., *Scritti 1953–1985* (pp. 702–730). Milan: Cortina, 2002.

Galimberti, U. (1996). La Nostra Origine In Fondo alla Grotta. *La Repubblica*, December 24.

Galimberti, U. (1997). Dialogo con il Caro Estinto. *La Repubblica*, January 21.

Geremek, B. (1973). Il Pauperismo nell'Era Preindustriale (secoli XIV-XVII). In: R. Romano and C. Vivanti (Eds.), op. cit., (pp. 669–698).

Geremek, B. (1986). *Poverty: A History*. A. Kolakowska (Trans.). Oxford (UK) and Malden, MA: Blackwell, 1997.

Giacanelli, F. (1975). Appunti per una Storia della Psichiatria in Italia, Introduzione. In: K. Dörner, op. cit., (pp. V–XXXII).

Giacanelli, F. (1980). Prefazione. In: Castel, R., op. cit., (pp. IX–XXI).

Gibelli, A. and Rugafiori, P. (Eds.) (1994). Storia d'Italia. Le Regioni dall'Unità ad Oggi. La Liguria. Turin: Einaudi.

Giroletti, A. (1996). *Morte e Psichiatria: fra Rappresentazione Simbolica e Realtà*, Master's Thesis in Psychiatry, University of Pavia. Not published.

Goffman, E. (1961). A*sylums. Essays on the Social Situation of Mental Patients and Other Inmates*. New York: Doubleday.

Gorer, G. (1956). The Pornography of Death. In: Id. (Ed.), *Death, Grief and Mourning* (pp. 192–199). New York: Doubleday, 1965.

Grinberg, L., and Grinberg, R. (1984). *Psychoanalytic Perspectives on Migration and Exile*. N. Festinger (Trans.).New Haven, CT: Yale University Press, 1989.

Guidoni, E. (1993). La Storia delle Piazze. In: A. Marino (Ed.), op.cit. (pp. 3–6).

Gutton, J.-P. (1974). *La Société et les Pauvres en Europe*. Paris: PUF.

Hochmann, J. (1971). *Pour une Psychiatrie Communautaire*. Paris: Seuil.

Hochmann, J. (1982). L'Or et le Cuivre. *Entrevues*, 4: 3–18.

Isnenghi, M. (1994). *L'Italia in Piazza. I Luoghi della Vita Pubblica dal 1948 ai Giorni Nostri*. Milan: Mondadori.

Izzo, E.M. (1983). Il Lavoro e gli Psicotici nelle Istituzioni. *Gli Argonauti, 17*: 147–155.

Izzo, E.M., and Lucchi, M. (1991). Il Significato del Lavoro nella Milieu-Thérapie della Schizofrenia. *Prospettive Psicoanalitiche nel Lavoro Istituzionale, 9*(2): 145–155.

Jaques, E. (1970). *Work, Creativity and Social Justice*. London: Heinemann.

Jervis, G. (1975). *Manuale Critico di Psichiatria*. Milan: Feltrinelli.

Jolivet, B. (1981). Travail et Thérapie de Réadaptation. In: *Encyclopédie Médico Chirurgicale*. Paris: Psychiatrie 37931, A 10, 10.

Jung, C.G. (1961). *Memories, Dreams, Reflections*. A. Jaffe (Ed.). C. Winston and R. Winston (Trans.). London: Vintage, 1989.

Juvenal (1991). S*atires I, III, X*. E. Courtney and N. Rudd (Eds.). Bristol: Bristol Classical Press.

Kleiner, J. (1970). On Nostalgia. *Bulletin of the Philadelphia Association for Psychoanalysis, 20*: 11–30.

Lader, M.H., and Herrington, R. (1990). *Biological Treatments in Psychiatry*. Oxford: Oxford University Press.

Levi, C. (1945). *Christ Stopped at Eboli*. F. Frenaye (Trans.). London: Penguin, 2000.

Levi, P. (1947). *Survival in Auschwitz: The Nazi Assault on Humanity*. S. Woolf (Trans.). New York: Collier Books, 1987. It originally appeared under the title *If This Is a Man*. London: The Orion Press, 1959.

Levi, P. (1978). *The Monkey's Wrench*. W. Weaver (Trans.). New York: Summit Books, 1986.

Liberman, R.P. (1988). *Psychiatric Rehabilitation of Chronic Mental Patients*. Washington: American Psychiatric Press.

LImentani, A. and Gaddini, E. (1992). A Psychianalytic Theiìory of Infalntile Experience. Conceptual and Clinical Refections (Italics). London and New York: Routledge.

Lindner, R.M. and R.V. Seliger, R.V. (Eds.) (1947). Handbook of Correctional Psychology. NewYork: Philosophical Library.

Lopez, D., and Zorzi Meneguzzo, L. (1989). Nostalgia. *Gli Argonauti, 40*: 3–8.

Lucas, U., (Ed.) (2004). Storia d'Italia, Annali 20 – L'Immagine Fotografica 1945–2000. Turin: Einaudi.

Lussana, P. (1994). La Composizione in Giorgione e il Tema della Natività e dell'Apprensione dell'Oggetto Estetico. *Psiche, 1*: 137–146.

Maccacaro, G. (1973). Il Bambino è dell'Ospedale? Seminario degli Studenti di Biometria e Statistica Medica dell'Università di Milano: Introduzione. In: Robertson, J., op. cit., (pp. XI–XL).

Magris, C. (1997). *Microcosms*. I. Halliday (Trans.). London: Harvill, 1999.

Mancuso, F. (1971). *Piazze d'Italia*. Milan: T.C.I.

Marazzi, F. (2015). *Le Città dei Monaci. Storia degli Spazi che Avvicinano a Dio*. Milan: Jaca Book.

Marino, A. (Ed.) (1993). *Le Piazze. Lo Spazio Pubblico dal Medioevo all'Età Contemporanea. Storia della Città, 54/55/56*. Milan: Electa.

Mas, M.V. (2019). *The Mad Women's Ball*. F. Wynne (Trans.). Ealing, London: Transworld Publishers, 2021.

Masini, U.M. (1908). Il Nuovo Manicomio Provinciale di Genova. *Liguria Medica, 2*, pp. 263–266.

Mastinu, A. (Ed.) (1982). Città, Salute Mentale, Psichiatria. Milan: Unicopli.

Maura, E., and Pisseri, P. (1991). *Le Strutture della Follia. Istituzioni e Società in Liguria dal XV° Secolo al XIX° Secolo*. Genoa: Sagep.

Maura, E., and Peloso, P.F. (1999). *Lo Splendore della Ragione. Storia della Psichiatria Ligure nell'Epoca del Positivismo*. 2 vol. Genoa: Sagep.

Meltzer, D. (1973). *Sexual States of Mind*. London: Phoenix, 2018.

Meltzer, D., and Harris Williams, M. (1988). *The Apprehension of Beauty: The Role of Aesthetic Conflict in Development, Art and Violence*. Perthshire: Clunie Press.

Menozzi, L. (1993). L'Idea di Piazza verso il 2000. In: A. Marino (Ed.), op. cit. (pp. 203–206).

Meriana, G. (1996). Presepe a Pratozanino. *Il Foglio, 4*: 1–7.

Molinari, A. (1994). La Città dei "Folli". Percorsi di Storia Sanitaria. In: A. Gibelli and P. Rugafiori (Eds.), op. cit., (pp. 420–432).

Natoli, S. (1995). Rimozione della Morte ed Epopea del Macabro. *La Morte e il Morire. Parole, Spirito e Vita, 32*: 341–358.

Nolen, W.A., and Haffmans, J. (1989). Treatment of Resistant Depression. Review on the Efficacy of Various Biological Treatments, specifically in Major Depression Resistant to Cyclic Antidepressants. *International Clinical Psychopharmacology, 4*(3): 217–228.

Oneroso Di Lisa, F. (1989). Nostalgia e Narcisismo. In: S. Vecchio (Ed.), op. cit. (pp. 41–56).

Ossicini, A. (1973). *Gli Esclusi e Noi*. Rome: Armando.

Papi, F. (1980). La Morte e il Simbolico. Una Tragedia Borghese. *Materiali Filosofici*, 3: 287–338.

Papuzzi, A. (1977). *Portami su Quello Che Canta*. Turin: Einaudi.

Parmiggiani, S. (Ed.), (2005). Il Volto della Follia. Cent'Anni di Immagini del Dolore. Geneva-Milan: Skira.

Pavan, F. (1984). La Paura di Attraversare e la Struttura Vissuta della Piazza. In: R. Rossi and F. Petrella (Eds.), *Psicoterapia delle Fobie* (pp. 253–260). Turin: Massaza & Sinchetto.

Pavan, F., and Schinaia, C. (1980). Appunti Clinici sulla Elettroshockterapia in Quattro Pazienti Melanconici. *Rassegna di Studi Psichiatrici*, 69(5): 1008–1030.

Pavan, F., and Zappalaglio, C. (1989). Il Problema dell'Osservare nel Rapporto con lo Psicotico Cronico. In: F. Petrella (Ed.), op. cit. (pp. 313–318).

Pedrinoni, I., and Tarantola, A. (1971). Contributo ad un'Impostazione Scientifica dell'Ergoterapia nelle Istituzioni Psichiatriche. *Neuropsichiatria*, 28(1–2): 279–297.

Peloso, P.F. (1992). Interventi In Tema di Ergoterapia sulla Stampa Medica Ligure Agli Inizi del Novecento. *Sanità, Scienza e Storia*, 1–2: 257–283.

Persad, F. (1990). Electroconvulsive Therapy in Depression. *Canadian Journal of Psychiatry*, 35: 175–181.

Petrella, F. (1969). *Sensory Deprivation*, Relazione e Coscienza. *Aut Aut*, 113: 78–83.

Petrella, F. (Ed.) (1986). *Psicoterapia dell'Anziano*. Turin: CST.

Petrella, F. (Ed.) (1989). *La Relazione Terapeutica nella Psicosi*. Turin: C.S.T.

Petrella, F. (1993a). Interno/esterno: Spazio vissuto e ambiente terapeutico. In: Id., *Turbamenti Affettivi e Alterazioni dell'Esperienza* (pp. 650–659). Milan: Cortina.

Petrella, F. (1993b). Sulla Riabilitazione in Psichiatria. In: Id., op. cit. (pp. 647–649).

Petrella, F. (1993c). Stati Confusionali e Metafore della Confusione. In: Id., op. cit. (pp. 180–203).

Petrella, F. (1993d). Ruoli e Aggressività in un Reparto Psichiatrico: Il Ciclo della Cronicizzazione. In: Id., op. cit. (pp. 431–436).

Petrella, F. (1993e). Istituzioni Fobiche e Istituzioni Ipocondriache. In: Id., op. cit. (pp. 480–483).

Petrella, F. (1993f). Istituzione Psichiatrica e Struttura della Personalità. In: Id., op. cit. (pp. 465–479).

Petrella, F. (1993g). Nostalgia: Tema con Variazioni. In: Id., op. cit. (pp. 391–403).

Petrella, F., Bezoari, M., Vender, S., and Weiss, G. (1978). Riflessioni su un'Esperienza Istituzionale con Pazienti Cronici: Crisi dell'"Équipe" e Significato della Dimissione. In: D. De Martis and M. Bezoari (Eds.), *Istituzione, Famiglia, "Équipe" Curante* (pp. 51–62). Milan: Feltrinelli.

Piccoli Catello, M. (Ed.), Il Presepe Napoletano. *La Collezione del Banco di Napoli*. Naples: Guida.

Pinel, Ph. (1801). *Medico-Philosophical Treatise on Mental Alienation*. G. Hickish, G. Healy, and L.C. Charland (Trans.). Hoboken (NJ): John Wiley & Sons, 2008.

Pisani, M. (Ed.) (1990). *Paolo Portoghesi. La Piazza come Luogo degli Sguardi*. Rome-Reggio Calabria: Gangemi.

Polach, J.-C., and Sivadon-Sabourin, D. (1976). *La Borde ou Le Droit à la Folie*. Paris: Calmann-Lévy.

Prete, A. (1992). L'Assedio della Lontananza. In: Id. (Ed.), *Nostalgia* (pp. 9–31). Milan: Cortina.

Prinzhorn, H. (1922). *Artistry of the Mentally Ill: A Contribution to the Psychology and Psychopathology of Configuration.* E. von Brockdorff (Trans.). Wien and New York: Springer-Verlag, 1995.

Proust, M. (1913). *In Search of Lost Time: Swann's Way, Vol. I.* C.K. Scott Moncrieff and T. Kilmartin (Trans.) and D.J. Enright (Rev.). New York: Modern Library, 1992.

Psichiatria Democratica (Ed.) (1975). *Bambini in Ospedale.* Rome: Bulzoni.

Psichiatria Democratica (1978). Documento Riassuntivo dei Lavori della Commissione sui Trattamenti Somatici in Psichiatria. Réseau Internazionale di Alternativa alla Psichiatria (Trieste 1977). *Fogli di informazione*, 44: 48–54.

Racamier, P.-C. (1970). *Le Psychanalyste sans Divan. La Psychanalyse et les Institutions de Soins Psychiatriques.* Paris: Payot.

Rank, O. (1909). *The Myth of the Birth of the Hero: A Psychological Exploration of Myth.* G.C. Richter and E.J. Lieberman (Trans.). Baltimore: Johns Hopkins University Press, 2004.

Rank, O. (1924). *The Trauma of Birth.* Translator's credit omitted. New York: Dover, 1993.

Richards, M.P.M. (1979). Effects on Development of Medical Interventions and Separation of Newborns from Their Parents. In: D. Shaffer and J. Dunn (Eds.), op. cit, (pp. 37–54).

Righetti, A., and Rotelli, F. (1990). Le Cooperative: Imprese Sociali tra Solidarietà e Produzione. *Fogli di Informazione*, 150: 29–32.

Riolfo Marengo, S. (1996). Prefazione. In: G. Buscaglia (Ed.), *I Presepi di Liguria* (pp. 9–11). Milan: Scheiwiller.

Ripert, P. (1956). *Les Origines de la Crèche Provençale et des Santons Populaires à Marseille.* Marseille: Tacussel.

Robertson, J. (1958). *Young Children in Hospitals.* New York: Basic Books. It. Translation: Bambini in Ospedale. L. Nahon, (It. Trans.). Milan: Feltrinelli, 1973.

Romano, C. (1990). Risocializzazione Psichiatrica e Lavoro – Parte Prima. *Quaderni Italiani di Psichiatria*, 9(3): 227–241.

Romano, C. (1992). Risocializzazione Psichiatrica e Lavoro – Parte Seconda. *Quaderni Italiani di Psichiatria*, 11(4): 299–328.

Romano, C. (1994). Risocializzazione Psichiatrica e Lavoro – Parte Terza. *Quaderni Italiani di Psichiatria*, 13(5): 221–243.

Romano, L. (1995). *Ho Sognato l'Ospedale.* Genoa: Il Melangolo.

Romano, R. and C. Vivanti, C. (Eds.) (1973). Storia d'Italia, Vol. 5. Turin: Einaudi.

Roussillon, R. (1988). Espaces et Pratiques Institutionnelles, le Débarras et l'Interstice. In: AA.VV., *L'Institution et les Institutions. Études Psychanalytiques* (pp. 17–176). Paris: Dunod.

Royal College of Psychiatrists (1977). Memorandum on the Use of Electroconvulsive Therapy. *British Journal of Psychiatry*, 131: 261–272.

Saraceno, B. (1982), Gli Spazi della Regola. In: A. Mastinu (Ed.), op. cit., (pp. 75–89).

Scala, A. (1975). Psicopatologia Urbana. *L'Ospedale Psichiatrico, numero monografico*, 43, fasc. 1–2.

Scaraffia, L. (2015). *Andare per Monasteri.* Bologna: Il Mulino.

Scarcella, M., Macrì, V., Adamo, P., and Bisignani, A. (1980). *Pericoloso a Sé e agli Altri.* Bari: De Donato.

Schinaia, C. (1983). La Morte e l'Ospedale. Tre Casi Clinici. *Devianza ed Emarginazione*, 5/6: 77–106.

Schinaia, C., and Soldi, G. (1985). La Crisi della Cartella Clinica come Strumento di Comunicazione in Psichiatria. *Prospettive Sociali e Sanitarie*, 15(12-13): 3–6.

Schinaia, C., Mazzoni, N., and Russo, F. (1985). L'Equivoco della Polarità Terapia-Assistenza. Note sull'Inserimento Lavorativo di Giovani Psicotici. *Il Ruolo Terapeutico*, 39: 8–13.

Schinaia, C., and Molteni, L. (1986). *Senectus ipsa mors?* Note sul Rapporto tra Vecchiaia e Morte. In: F. Petrella (Ed.), op. cit. (pp. 109–114).

Schinaia, C., Borchini, S., Cagnana, O., and Repetto, P. (1991). Ritornare in Manicomio. *Prospettive Sociali e Sanitarie*, 21(15): 12–16.

Schinaia, C., Barisone, M., Ferro, M., and Ciammella, L. (1992). Itinerari Narrativi attraverso la Fotografia Psichiatrica. *Prospettive Psicoanalitiche nel Lavoro Istituzionale*, 10(3): 291–297.

Schinaia, C., and Cagnana, O. (1993). Ritornare in Manicomio (2). *Prospettive Sociali e Sanitarie*, 23(12): 18–19.

Schinaia, C. Barisone, M., Ferro, M., and Ciammella, L. (1994). Dallo Sguardo al Racconto. Percorsi Narrativi attraverso l'Anamnesi Psichiatrica. *Gli Argonauti*, 61: 163–170.

Schinaia, C., Barisone, M., and Fato, M. (1995). Falso Movimento. Sugli Aspetti Relazionali della Discinesia Tardiva. *Gli Argonauti*, 66: 255–261.

Schinaia, C., and Marcenaro, C. (1996). Ritornare in Manicomio (3). *Prospettive Sociali e Sanitarie*, 26(3): 15–18.

Schinaia, C. (1998a). *Il Cantiere delle Idee. Le Feste nell'ex Ospedale psichiatrico di Cogoleto*. Genoa: La Clessidra. Reprinted Rome: Vecchiarelli, 2023.

Schinaia, C. (1998b). Che Cosa ci Fa uno Psicoanalista in un Ex Manicomio? A Piero Leonardi e Dario De Martis. In: L. Pesce and P.F. Peloso (Eds.), *180 Vent'Anni Dopo* (pp. 97–111). Albisola Superiore (Sv): La Redancia.

Schinaia, C. (2001). Immagini della Follia tra Memoria e Progetto. Saggio Introduttivo. In: Lucas, U., *Altri Sguardi* (pp. 5–15). Rome: T-Scrivo.

Schinaia, C. (2004). Fotografia e Psichiatria. In: U. Lucas, (Ed.), op. cit., (pp. 459–476).

Schinaia, C. (2005). Chiaroscuri. Sui Rapporti tra Fotografia e Psichiatria. In: S. Parmiggiani (Ed.), op. cit., (pp. 33–46).

Schinaia, C. (2019). *Psychoanalysis and Architecture. The Inside and the Outside*. London and New York: Routledge.

Schinaia, C. (2023a). Morire in Ospedale. In: G. De Intinis (Ed.), *op. cit.* (pp. 143–184).

Schinaia, C. (2023b). Alcune Note sul Lavoro in Psichiatria. In: G. De Intinis (Ed.), op. cit. (pp. 185–196).

Sediari, F., Giacanelli, F., and Rotondi, A. (1966). Le Esigenze Spaziali del Malato di Mente. In AA.VV., *Conference Proceedings "Aspetti Sociopsicopatologici di Architettura ed Urbanistica," Treviso* (pp. 40–45).

Senn, M. (Ed.) (1949). *Problems of Infancy and Childhood: Transactions of the Third Conference on Problems of Infancy and Childhood*. New York: Josiah Macy Jr.

Shaffer, D. and J. Dunn, J. (Eds.) (1979). The First Year of Life: Psychological and Medical Implications of Early Experience. Chichester: Wiley.

Sindacati Confederali (1974). *Libro Bianco sui Manicomi Genovesi*. Genoa: A.T.A. Retrieved from https://www.imfi-ge.org/wp/wpcontent/uploads/2019/12/Libro-bianco-manicomi-genovesi.pdf.

Slavich, A., and Jervis Comba, L. (1973). Il Lavoro Rende Liberi? Commento a Due Assemblee di Comunità dell'Ospedale Psichiatrico di Gorizia. In: F. Basaglia (Ed.), *Che Cos'È la Psichiatria?* (pp. 69–152). Turin: Einaudi.

Sohn, L. (1983). Nostalgia. *The International Journal of Psychoanalysis, 64*(2): 203–211.

Solnit, A., and Stark, M. (1961). Mourning and the Birth of a Defective Child. *Psychoanalytical Study of the Child, 16*(1): 523–537.

Sommariva, G. (1993). Aspetti Tecnologici e Scenografici del Presepe Genovese. In: Soprintendenza per i Beni Artistici e Storici della Liguria (Ed.), op. cit., (pp. 58–73).

Soprintendenza per i Beni Artistici e Storici della Liguria, (dir.) (1993). Venite Adoremus. Note sul Presepe Genovese. Genoa: Tormena.

Spinelli, E. (1995). *Se il Matto Non Sparisce ... Dalla Dipendenza all'Interdipendenza nel Lavoro dei Servizi.* Milan: FrancoAngeli.

Spitz, R.A. (1965). *The First Year of Life: A Psychoanalytic Study of Normal and Deviant Development of Object Relations.* New York: International University Press, 1992.

Stanton, A.H., and Schwartz, M.S. (1954). *The Mental Hospital.* New York: Basic Books.

Starobinski, J. (1984). Préface. In: Prinzhorn H. *Expressions de la Folie: Dessins, Peintures, Sculptures d'Asile* (pp. VII–XVI). Paris: Gallimard.

Stefanucci, A. (1961) s.v. Presepe. In: *Enciclopedia dello Spettacolo.* Rome: Le Maschere, 1961.

Steegmuller, F. (Ed. and Trans.) (1980). *The Letters of Gustave Flaubert (1830–1857),* 2 Vol. Cambridge (MA) and London: Belknap/Harvard University Press.

Steiner, J. (1993). *Psychic Retreats: Pathological Organizations in Psychotic, Neurotic, and Borderline Patients.* London and New York: Routledge.

Stella, S. (1983). *Lavoro Interno e Lavoro Esterno. Premesse ad una Psicoanalisi del Lavoro.* Turin: CST.

Stern, D. (1985). *The Interpersonal World of the Infant.* New York: Basic Books.

Sullivan, H.S. (1940). Conceptions of Modern Psychiatry. *Psychiatry, 3*: 1–117.

Tagliabue, L. (1993). La Riabilitazione. In: F. Asioli et al. (Eds.), op. cit. (pp. 213–237).

Tanzi, E. (1905). *Trattato delle Malattie Mentali,* 2 Vol. Milan: S.E.I.

Teobaldi, P. (2007). *Il Mio Manicomio.* Rome: e/o.

Todd, E. (1830). *Report of a Committee of the Connecticut Medical Society, Respecting an Asylum for Inebriates: With the Resolutions of the Society, Adopted at Their Annual Meeting.* New Haven: Hezekiah Howe.

Tosatti, B. (Ed.) (1998). *Figure dell'Anima. Arte Irregolare in Europa.* Catalog of the Exhibitions in Pavia and Genoa. Milan: Mazzotta.

Totò (De Curtis, A.) (1989). *A Livella. Poesie Napoletane.* Naples: Fausto Fiorentino.

Tuke, S. (1964). *Description of the Retreat, an Institution near York for Insane Persons of the Society of Friends.* London: Dawson's of Pall Mall.

Turner, V. (1969). *The Ritual Process: Structure and Anti-Structure.* London and New York: Routledge, 1996.

Van Gennep, A. (1909). *The Rites of Passage.* M.B. Vizedom and G.L. Caffee (Trans.). Chicago: University of Chicago Press, 1961.

Vecchio, S. (Ed.) (1989). *Nostalgia.* Bergamo: Lubrina.

Vender, S. (1987). Le Ricerche sui Giornali e la Malattia Mentale in Italia. In: D. De Martis et al. (Eds.), op. cit. (pp. 19–42).

Walter, B. (2002). Hermann Simon – Psychiatriereformer, Sozialdarwinist, Nationalsozialist? [Hermann Simon--Reformer of Psychiatry, Social Darwinist, and National Socialist?]. *Nervenarzt*, 73(11): 1047–1054.

Warner, R. (1985). *Recovery from Schizophrenia: Psychiatry and Political Economy.* London and New York: Routledge.

Winnicott, D.W. (1949). Birth Memories, Birth Trauma and Anxiety. In: Id., *Collected Papers: Through Paediatrics to Psycho-Analysis.* London: Tavistock, 1958. Reprinted as *Trough Paediatrics to Psychoanalysis: Collected Papers* (pp. 174-193). London: Hogarth Press, 1975.

Winnicott, D. W. (1951). Transitional Objects and Transitional Phenomena. In: Id., Through Paediatrics to Psycho-Analysis: Collected Papers. London: Tavistock, 1958. Reprinted as Trough Paediatrics to Psychoanalysis: Collected Papers (pp. 229–242). London: Hogarth Press, 1975.

Winnicott, D.W. (1965). *The Maturational Processes and the Facilitating Environment.* London: Hogarth Press.

Winnicott, D.W. (1984). *Deprivation and Delinquency.* M. Davis, R. Shepherd, and C. Winnicott (Eds.). London and New York: Routledge.

Winnicott, D.W. (1971). *Playing and Reality.* London: Tavistock. Reprinted London and New York: Routledge, 1991.

Zappalaglio, C., and Pavan, F. (1986). E. Kraepelin come Maestro. Critica alla Modalità Perversa dell'Osservare. *Gli Argonauti*, 30: 223–238.

Index

Pages in *italics* refer to figures.